Back

to

Brilliant

ABOUT THE AUTHOR

Duncan Lawler is a senior chartered physiotherapist, a licensed physical therapist in the USA, manual handling instructor, CPR instructor, a qualified acupuncturist who lectures for the British Medical Acupuncture society, he is an international speaker, an author of several books but most importantly of all, he is a person just like you, who has experienced back pain and understands the pain, the fear, the worry, the disappointment that you are going through.

'If you change the way you look at things – the things you look at change'
Dr. Wayne Dyer

Author's Acknowledgements:

Patrick Cumiskey for all your support, motivation and help.

Eileen McCormack for her eye for detail.

For every patient that ever thanked me, your gratitude makes it worthwhile.

Table Of Contents:

CHAPTER 1: BACK TO BASICS

Introduction:

The human body was built for movement, for physical activity, with speed and precision being significant factors. Our ancestors chased after animals for meat, climbed trees for fruit, walked miles in search of grain. Mobility in all joints was maintained and the stronger muscles were used to propel the body and lift whatever weight that was required to be carried. Squatting was the position of choice.

In cultures where similar customs remain practiced to this day, there is very little incidence of low back pain or slipped disk. Technologies have been to our benefit but also our detriment as we no longer present as active or mobile as bodies were designed to be. The result is that back pain is an affliction which affects about 80% of the population in Western countries and that probably includes you!

Knowledge is power and the following chapter details what you need to know about your back in simple English, where medical jargon is used - it will be explained clearly.

Structure of the Back:

The spine is made up of a column of bones called vertebrae, topped by the skull and based on the pelvis (or hips). Cushioned between the vertebrae is a disc, which acts as a shock absorber.

The disk is made up of an outer ring of cartilage and a jelly-like centre. At the back of the spine are small joints between the vertebrae and these are held together by ligaments.

The spine is strengthened and made flexible by a group of muscles. This structure changes your back from a rigid rod into a flexible spine.

Functions of the Back:

The spine carries the weight of the top half of the body and transfers it to the pelvis. The spine includes the spinal cord. This cord is connected directly to the brain. The cord is connected to the nerves between each vertebrae and these control the movement of the trunk, arms and legs and convey all sensations.

Discs cushioned between the vertebrae, bound by ligaments and muscles allow movement and flexibility. Without discs the spine would be like a bamboo and we could not bend forward, backwards, sideways or look behind us.

DEFINING BACK PAIN:

Types of back pain

Lower back pain

This is the most prevalent type of back pain with around 8 out of 10 people affected at some time in their lives. The lower back is defined as the area between the bottom of the ribcage and the top of the legs. Symptoms range from tension and stiffness to pain and soreness. Most people's back pain is described as non-specific, meaning it is caused by structures in the back as opposed to rare conditions such as cancer or a fracture.

Lower back pain is often triggered by everyday activities such as bending awkwardly, lifting incorrectly, and standing for long periods of time, slouching when sitting and driving for long periods without taking breaks

Buttocks and legs (sciatica)

Sciatica is pain caused by irritation or compression of the sciatic nerve. The sciatic nerve is the longest nerve in your body and runs from the back of your pelvis, through your buttocks, and all the way down both legs, ending at your feet.

When something compresses or irritates the sciatic nerve, it can cause a pain that radiates out from your lower back and travels down your leg to your calf. This can be mild to very painful.

The most common cause of sciatica is a slipped disc. This occurs when one of the discs that sit between the vertebrae is ruptured.

For persistent sciatica, you may be advised to try a structured exercise program under the supervision of a physiotherapist. In rare cases, surgery may be needed to control the symptoms.

Sciatica is the name given to any sort of pain that is caused by irritation or compression of the sciatic nerve.

Symptoms of Sciatica

Sciatica is different to general back pain; the pain of sciatica hardly affects the back at all but radiates out from the lower back, down the buttocks and into one or both of the legs, right down to the calf.

Sciatic pain can range from being mild to very painful and can last for weeks or months. If it lasts for more than six weeks, it is considered persistent (chronic) sciatica.

Other symptoms

If you have sciatica, you may also experience the following symptoms around your legs and feet:

- Numbness
- Tingling
- Muscle weakness
- Loss of tendon reflexes

A slipped disc is the most common identified cause of sciatica, but in some cases there is no obvious cause.

Other causes

Less commonly, sciatica may be caused by:

- Infection
- Injury
- A growth within the spine, such as a tumor

Cauda Equina Syndrome

Cauda equina syndrome is a rare but serious condition that can cause sciatica. The cauda equina is the bundle of nerves that leads out from the end of the spinal cord. Cauda equina syndrome occurs when these nerves are compressed and damaged.

It can eventually lead to paralysis if left untreated.

One of the warning signs of cauda equina syndrome is suddenly losing control of your bladder or bowels. If this happens, see a doctor immediately.

Other Symptoms include:

- Lower back pain
- Numbness in your groin
- Paralysis of one or both legs
- Rectal pain
- Bowel disturbance
- Inability to pass urine or incontinence
- Pain in the inside of your thighs

You should seek medical assistance immediately if you develop these symptoms. Visit your GP or the accident and emergency (A&E) department of your nearest hospital. If cauda equina syndrome is not promptly treated, the nerves to your bladder and bowel can become permanently damaged.

Slipped (herniated) disc

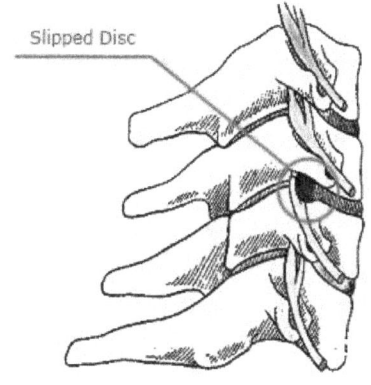

Slipped Disc

A slipped (or herniated) disc is the most common identified cause of sciatica. Your spine is made up of vertebrae, discs and nerves. Vertebrae are the blocks of bone that make up the structure of your spine and protect the nerves. The vertebrae are supported and cushioned by discs. The discs are made from a tough, fibrous case that contains a softer gel-like substance. A slipped disc occurs when the outer part of the disc ruptures (splits), allowing the gel inside to bulge and protrude outwards between the vertebrae. When this presses against the sciatic nerve, it can cause sciatica.

As a person gets older the discs start to become harder, tougher and more brittle. Repeated strain on the back means there is a greater chance of a hardened disc splitting and rupturing.

Most people who have a slipped disc experience pain which usually begins in the lower back before sometimes spreading to other parts of the body.

However, some people with a slipped disc do not have any obvious symptoms. This is usually because the part of the disc that bulges out is small or does not press on nerves or spinal cord.

If the slipped disc presses on any of the other nerves that run down your spinal cord, your symptoms may include:

- Muscle paralysis (weakness)
- Muscle spasms - where your muscles contract tightly and painfully
- Loss of bladder control (urinary incontinence)

Muscle spasms and paralysis tend to occur in your arms, legs and buttocks. The pain you experience when a disc presses on a nerve is often worse when you put pressure on the nerve. This can happen when you cough, sneeze or sit down.

What causes a slipped disc?

A slipped disc occurs when the outer case of the disc ruptures (splits), resulting in the gel inside bulging and protruding out of the disc.

The damaged disc can put pressure on the whole spinal cord or on a single nerve root. This means that a slipped disc can cause pain both in the area of the protruding disc and in the area of the body that is controlled by the nerve that the disc is pressing on.

It is not always clear what causes a disc to break down, although age is a common factor in many cases. As you get older, your spinal discs start to lose their water content, making them less flexible and more likely to rupture.

There are a number of other factors that can put increased pressure and strain on your spine. These include:

- Bending awkwardly
- Jobs that involve heavy or awkward lifting
- Jobs that involve lots of sitting, particularly driving
- Smoking
- Being overweight
- Weight-bearing sports, such as weight lifting
- A traumatic injury to your back, such as a fall or car accident

Situations such as these can weaken the disc tissue and can sometimes lead to a slipped disc.

Diagnosing a slipped disc

Your GP will usually be able to diagnose a slipped disc from your symptoms and medical history. They may also carry out a physical examination to test:

- Reflexes
- Muscles strength
- Walking ability
- Sensation in your limbs
- Straight leg-raising test

While you are lying flat, your GP will slowly raise each of your legs, one at a time, to see if it causes any pain or discomfort in your legs or back. This is known as the straight leg raise test or SLR.

Most people with a slipped disc will not be able to raise their leg more than two thirds of the way up without feeling tingling, numbness and pain.

Further tests

If your symptoms do not ease after 4-6 weeks, further tests may be required to rule out other conditions and investigate the size and position of the slipped disc.

Some of the tests that you may have are described below.

Magnetic resonance imaging scan

A magnetic resonance imaging (MRI) scan uses a strong magnetic field and radio waves to produce detailed images of the inside of your body.

MRI scans are effective at showing the position and size of a slipped disc. They can also pinpoint the affected nerves.

Computerized tomography scan

A computerized tomography (CT) scan uses a series of X-rays to scan parts of your body. A computer is used to build up detailed images of your body.

This produces cross-sectional images of your spinal column and the structures that surround it. Similar to an MRI scan, a CT scan can pinpoint a slipped disc, although it is often not as effective.

Discography

A discography is a test where a special dye is injected into the disc in your spine.

An X-ray will then be taken to show how the dye has spread around your back. The image will reveal any tears or leaks from your disc.

Spinal Stenosis

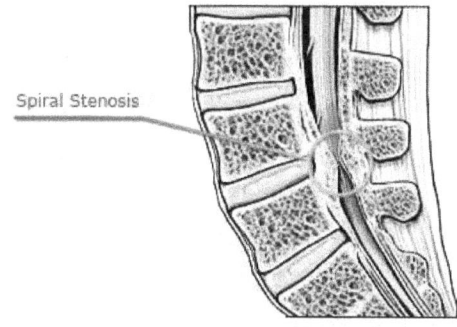

Spiral Stenosis

Spinal stenosis is the narrowing of nerve passages in the spine. It occurs when the bones, ligaments or discs of the spine squash the nerves of the spine (usually the sciatic nerve) causing pain, usually in the lower back and legs. It usually affects people in late middle age and older.

Causes of spinal stenosis include:

- Age-related changes in the spine
- Changes in the ligaments of the spine
- Diseases of the bone, such as Paget's disease

Low Back Pain Causes

Back pain is a symptom. There are over one hundred accepted causes of low back pain with wear and tear being the most common cause of pain.

Wear and tear can affect the discs and the joints between the vertebrae. The cartilage or smooth covering of the joint becomes roughened and worn with spikes of bone growing out from the side of the joint. This prevents the joint from moving freely and leads to stiffness.

The discs may become thinner and the spikes of bone may press on nerve roots as they leave the spinal canal causing pain or such sensations as pins and needles or numbness.

Wear and tear changes in the spine can be noticed from as early as twenty-five years of age or even younger if there has been an earlier injury. There are a number of causes of backache due to excessive wear and tear - for example an earlier injury, heavy physical work over a long period, overweight and lack of fitness.

Other common causes of back pain involve disease or injury to the muscles, bones, and/or nerves of the spine. Pain arising from abnormalities of organs within the abdomen, pelvis, or chest may also be felt in the back. This is called referred pain.

Many disorders within the abdomen, such as appendicitis, aneurysms, kidney diseases, kidney infection, bladder infections, pelvic infections, and ovarian disorders, prostate problems among others, can cause pain referred to the back. Normal pregnancy can cause back pain in many ways, including stretching ligaments within the pelvis, irritating nerves, and straining the low back.

Nerve root syndromes are those that produce symptoms of nerve impingement (a nerve is directly irritated), often due to a herniation (or bulging) of the disc between the lower back bones. Sciatica is an example of nerve root impingement. Impingement pain tends to be sharp, affecting a specific area, and associated with numbness in the area of the leg that the affected nerve supplies.

Herniated discs develop as the spinal discs degenerate or grow thinner. The jelly-like central portion of the disc bulges out of the central cavity and pushes against a nerve root. Intervertebral discs begin to degenerate by the third decade of life. Herniated discs are found in one-third of adults older than twenty years of age. Only three percent of these, however, produce symptoms of nerve impingement.

Discs lose moisture and volume with age, which decreases the disc height. Even minor trauma under these circumstances can cause inflammation and nerve root impingement, which can produce classic sciatica without disc rupture.

Spinal disc degeneration coupled with disease in joints of the low back can lead to spinal-canal narrowing (spinal stenosis). These changes in the disc and the joints produce symptoms and can be seen on an X-ray.

A person with spinal stenosis may have pain radiating down both lower extremities while standing for a long time or walking even short distances.

Strained Muscles (Lumbago)

Muscles are strained by overloading. This is usually caused by a sudden or unexpected movement, like catching a heavy falling object. Muscles are easily strained if you are not fit, or do not warm up before taking exercise, or when muscles are fatigued.

Strained Ligaments

Ligaments prevent excessive movement at the joints of the spine. They can be injured when a joint is stretched to its limit and held there too long or repeated too often.

Musculoskeletal pain syndromes that produce low back pain include myo-fascial pain syndromes and fibromyalgia.

Myo-fascial pain is characterized by pain and tenderness over localized areas (trigger points), loss of range of motion in the involved muscle groups, and pain radiating in a characteristic distribution but restricted to a peripheral nerve. Relief of pain is often reported when the involved muscle group is stretched.

Fibromyalgia results in widespread pain and tenderness throughout the body. Generalized stiffness, fatigue, and muscle aches are reported.

Infections of the bones (osteomyelitis) of the spine are an uncommon cause of low back pain.

Non-infectious inflammation of the spine (spondylitis) can cause stiffness and pain in the spine that is particularly worse in the morning. Ankylosing spondylitis typically begins in adolescents and young adults.

Tumors, possibly cancerous, can be a source of skeletal pain.

Inflammation of nerves from the spine can occur with infection of the nerves with the herpes zoster virus that causes shingles. This can occur in the thoracic area to cause upper back pain or in the lumbar area to cause low back pain.

As can be seen from the extensive, but not all inclusive, list of possible causes of low back pain, it is important to have a thorough medical evaluation to guide possible diagnostic tests.

Low Back Pain Symptoms

- Pain in the lumbosacral area (lower part of the back) is the primary symptom of low back pain.

- The pain may radiate down the front, side, or back of your leg, or it may be confined to the low back.

- The pain may become worse with activity.

- Occasionally, the pain may be worse at night or with prolonged sitting such as on a long car trip.

- You may have numbness or weakness in the part of the leg that receives its nerve supply from a compressed nerve possibly causing an inability to plantar flex the foot resulting in being unable to stand on your toes or bring your foot downward. This occurs when the first sacral nerve is compressed or injured.

- Another example would be the inability to raise your big toe upward. This results when the fifth lumbar nerve is compromised.

MYTHS AND MISUNDERSTANDINGS ABOUT BACK PAIN

Myth: Back Pain and Back Problems Won't Happen to Me

Fact: Approximately eight out of ten people will experience back pain at some point in their lifetime. So, unfortunately, the fact is that most people do experience back pain and back problems at some point in their lives.

Myth: Bad Back Pain Can Result in Paralysis

Fact: The spinal cord ends in the upper part of the lower back (between the first and second lumbar vertebrae). Further down the low back there are only nerve roots, which are very tough structures. In most cases, a great deal of back pain does not usually indicate a back problem that could lead to paralysis. Examples of rare cases where paralysis may be a risk include spine tumors, spinal infections and unstable spine fractures.

Myth: Severe Back Pain Correlates to the Level of Back Damage

Fact: With acute pain, the level of pain correlates to the level of damage (e.g. if you touch a hot iron, you will immediately feel a great deal of pain). However, with chronic back pain (greater than six weeks), the amount of pain does not typically correlate the amount of damage.

Myth: I am Physically Active, So I Shouldn't Get Back Pain

Fact: While it is true that well-conditioned individuals are less likely to have an episode of back pain than sedentary individuals, back pain can affect all people regardless of the level of activity. Some sports are more likely to cause back pain, such as golf, volleyball and gymnastics. In all cases, however, the back should be considered a priority in conditioning, because it creates a stable platform from which the arms and legs work.

Myth: If I have back pain and back problems when I am young, it will get worse as I age.

Fact: The incidence of back pain is actually highest between the ages of thirty-five and fifty-five. After age fifty-five, people usually have less pain - especially discogenic pain (back pain or other pain or symptoms caused by disc problems). While disc degeneration is a natural part of the aging process, it is not always accompanied by pain.

Myth: An MRI scan or other diagnostic test is needed to diagnose my back problem.

Fact: Most health professionals can develop a successful treatment approach based on a thorough medical history and physical examination. Only specific symptom patterns in a minority of cases indicate the need for an MRI scan or other sophisticated tests. Typically, an MRI scan is used when patients are not responding to appropriate back pain treatment.

Myth: The abnormality/back problems on my MRI scan needs to be cured.

Fact: An abnormality that is seen on an imaging test (MRI, CT scan) does not necessarily cause back pain or other symptoms. In fact, the vast majority of people who never have had an episode of low back pain will have abnormalities (such as a herniated disc or degenerative disc) on an imaging test. For patients experiencing low back pain, 92%-96% can be treated successfully without back surgery.

Myth: My discs go back when manipulated my spine pops?

NO: When your spine pops, it is simply a release of gas from the joints.

Your discs never move, the middle part simply bulges. 'Slipped disc' is simply a layman's term for a bulging or herniated disc.

Think about what happens when you crack your knuckles. Prior to cracking your knuckles, move your fingers around. Do any of your fingers appear out of alignment? Despite the fact that your knuckles are clearly in alignment, you can still crack them. That's because you are simply releasing gas from the joint when you distract or separate the joints. Try to pop your knuckles again within twenty minutes of your initial cracking and you'll find that you are unable to produce any noise. This is because the gas has not had adequate time to assimilate back into the joint fluid where it can be released again. The same phenomenon occurs in your back. Cracking your back has little to do with the alignment of your spine.

Myth: Cracking my back will make my problems disappear

Fact: In some cases, cracking your back can indeed significantly reduce your symptoms. The reason for this is that it can cause muscles to relax that may be in spasm or causing compression on sensitive tissues. At other times, however, cracking your back will lead to increased pain. It all depends on what tissues are damaged. Cracking your back requires all the tissues around the joint to be maximally stretched. If some of these tissues are injured, then you can count on your pain being increased after having your spine manipulated. It is important to remember that the spine is made up of the same exact tissues as the rest of your body. If you sprained your ankle, is there anything that you think could be done to magically make your ankle instantly return to normal?

By the same token you should not expect any particular treatment for your spine to instantly alleviate your symptoms. Spraining your back is no different than spraining your ankle. Tissues are damaged and must be given a chance to heal. Any treatment you receive to your back, or any other body part, has the same goal. Treatments are designed to remove barriers that may be impeding your body from healing itself. It is the body that must do the healing not the practitioner. Until your body heals itself your problems will remain.

Myth: If my hip is out of place, will this cause back pain?

Fact: Many patients state that they have been told that their back pain is related to their hips being out of joint. This is most likely never the case. Dislocating a hip requires a tremendous amount of force and results in a tremendous amount of pain. You would be unable to walk and the hip would need to be manipulated into place immediately by a physician. The reason your back pain decreases following a manipulation (popping) of the hip is that your hips are connected to your pelvis which in turn connects to your spine. When your hips receive a strong pull, the force will also be directed to your spine. This will cause the spine to stretch which produces a similar effect to manipulating or cracking the spine.

As additional evidence, patients that are diagnosed with hip related back pain are given this diagnosis based on the fact that one leg is shorter than the other. The leg length diagnosis is given based on external observation (i.e. simply looking at leg lengths visually). This is highly inaccurate. The only way to truly discern a leg length discrepancy is through x-rays. The next best method would be to utilize a tape measure on bony prominences between the pelvis and ankle.

Many people are born with differences between their leg lengths. If a person is born with one leg longer than the other, no amount of manipulation will cause this to change. Obviously if one leg is physically shorter than the other one this is perfectly normal for that particular individual and in no way indicates abnormal pathology of any part of the body.

CHAPTER 2: Treatment

Back pain and treatment is a topic that everyone has an opinion on, and every opinion appears to be different.

Even though back pain is an incredibly common condition, huge confusion surrounds the problem both for patients and healthcare professionals.

In the majority of cases, the exact source of the pain remains unknown. Healthcare providers show considerable disagreement as to specific diagnoses and appropriate treatment plans. These two problems result in the possibility of obtaining a wide variety of diagnosis and treatment recommendations as you search for answers to your back pain. In fact, the more you search, the more confused you may feel.

Unfortunately, many people with back pain are treated as if their pain is imaginary or exaggerated. Over the years one has seen patients whose pain has been dismissed so often by friends and family that they feel the need to convince me of their pain when they first attend.

To make matters more challenging, in back pain cases there is often very little or no physical evidence to explain the pain. Back pain sufferers go from one therapist to the next, searching for explanations. They struggle through one unnecessary evaluation after another and never-ending treatments. Sometimes patients are actually harmed by well-meaning but poorly informed healthcare professionals (or not so professional) who treat back pain incorrectly.

So let's now return to back to basics and revisit the anatomy of your back. Your lower back consists of six structures.

These are the:
- Vertebrae
- Joint
- Nerves
- Muscles,
- Ligaments and
- Disc.

You can injure or damage any one of these components. These components however work in conjunction with each other; therefore a problem with one component will affect another. Hence lower back pain is incredibly complex as not only does it require diagnosing the structure causing the problem but also knowing what or how the other structures are affected.

All back problems consist of an injury to one or more of these structures. This is why some people spend forever finding a 'cure' with unfortunately no success or how some people have surgery but remain in pain afterwards.

Improving and managing back pain is about calculating what degree each component is responsible for the pain.
If the problem were a joint for example - the solution would be manual therapy, this could involve manipulating the segment or gently mobilizing the segment.
If the problem were a nerve - the solution might be electrotherapy, electro acupuncture or acupuncture itself as these modalities have an effect on neural structures.

If the problem were a muscle - the solution perhaps could be massage, myo-fascial release, trigger point needling or ultrasound as these methods alter muscle physiology.

If the problem were a ligament - an approach could be passive stretching, exercise therapy, ultrasound or gentle mobilizations of the affected structure.

If the problem were bone - this may require surgery or medication.

If the problem was a herniated disc of severe magnitude - this may require surgery and medication.

The complex issue is that the problem is never purely exclusively one structure but a combination of structures, all which may not contribute equally to the pain.

There is no substitute for having extensive knowledge of every aspect of treatment and experience.

An additional contributing factor is that of circulation and this adds to the complexity of the case. No two back problems are the same and every person responds uniquely to different treatments. Symptoms shared between two people who appear similar may actually be from two completely different problems.

Before you embark on your quest for successful treatment remember, doctors identify no specific structural problem in the majority of back pain cases. Surgery is rarely necessary in order to become pain free.

Effective treatment is possible without a specific diagnosis. Structural abnormalities (such as a herniated disc) often have nothing to do with your pain.

How is my back treated?

Physiotherapy: Your doctor may recommend physiotherapy for your back pain. Examples of this treatment include special exercises, manual therapy or manipulation, deep tissue massage, and electrotherapy.

Medications: Doctors use a variety of medications in treating back pain including analgesics (painkillers), anti-inflammatory, muscle relaxants among others.

Braces and Corsets: Braces and corsets restrict motion, provide support, may decrease pain, and correct posture in the lower back area. General back supports are available without a prescription. Your doctor or physiotherapist should always guide your use of a back brace.

Exercise: Your doctor or physiotherapist may recommend different types of exercise programs for back pain, including lumbar stabilization, cardiovascular conditioning and others:

Spinal epidural steroid and nerve blocks: These treatments involve injecting certain medicines into a particular area of the spinal canal to help with back pain and nerve irritation.

Trigger-point injection therapy: This treatment involves injecting a small amount of anesthetic pain-killer into trigger points, the areas of a muscle that seem to trigger pain in a given region of the body.

Pain Management: Pain management combines a variety of approaches - psychological approaches, medicine, exercise and working with family members to address your pain problem.

Stress management and posture: Stress management such as relaxation training, yoga, and thought analysis can help with back pain problems. Addressing your posture in your work or home environment can also be an important part of your treatment.

Acupuncture: An ancient Chinese medicine approach in which small needles that pierce the skin are placed at specific points to cause healing and other benefits such as pain relief.

Chiropractic: This treatment influences the body's nervous system and ability to heal through adjustments of the spine, muscles and joints.

Magnet Therapy: This therapy involves the application of a magnetic field (produced by a magnet or electrical device) to a body part. Magnets have long been thought to have healing properties.

Mind-Body approaches: A number of different approaches can promote the body's own ability to heal itself and increase the mind's power over the body.

Yoga: A system of health that uses physical postures, breathing exercises and meditation to relieve suffering and enhance overall well-being.

Who and how to choose?

- Do your research and ask questions.
- What risks or potential side effects are associated with this treatment?
- At what point in the treatment will you and your practitioner know whether the treatment is working?
- What is a reasonable treatment trial (for example, how many sessions)?

- Beware of quick fixes. If you have chronic back pain, you may be more susceptible to claims for a quick fix due to your frustration over the ongoing pain and you are longing for relief.

  o What is the therapist's qualification?

  o Determining the treating practitioner's professional degree is important.

  o Where did they train?

  o Know where your therapist/doctor did his or her training in terms of medical school education and training.

  o To what medical and professional societies do they belong?

Ask about the types of medical and/or professional societies in which your practitioner has membership, because this information can give you an idea of his or her treatment focus. Membership in specialized societies usually indicates that the healthcare professional is obtaining continuing education.

  o How long have they been practicing?

  o Do they have special training in treating back pain problems?

  o What percentage of patients do they see with back pain problems?

  o Get a referral from a dependable source.

  o Will they work with your doctor?

The practitioner needs to be willing to work and communicate with your doctor. Although communication may not always be necessary, you need to know that your practitioner would contact your doctor if he/she felt it was necessary.

'Can you tell me how low long and how often I should expect to be treated?'

This question is appropriate for anyone providing you with treatment. You should have an idea as to how long and how often you will be treated based upon the practitioners' work with patients similar to you.

HOME REMEDIES

You can manage and treat most episodes of back pain on your own but there are a few warning signs that mean you should head straight to the doctor for evaluation. These are discussed in greater detail in Chapter 8.

- You can't control your bowel or bladder

- Your legs are weak or you experience foot drop

- Your back pain awakens you at night

- You experience a significant trauma such as a car accident or a fall.

- Your back pain is excruciating.

Using home remedies.

If your back pain appears to be worsening as you use any of the home remedies, visit your doctor.

<u>Hints and tips</u>.

- Wear a brace or corset

- Apply a topical anti-irritant to sore muscles

- Have your muscles LIGHTLY massaged and stretched

- Engage in deep breathing

Let pain be your guide. Listen to the pain signal and stop what you are doing. If you are in the middle of a sporting activity you may want to stop it after some cooling down movements such as stretching or gentle walking.

If severe - bed rest but only for two to three days. Extended bed rest for back pain promotes muscle weakness, decreased flexibility, stomach and bowel problems and ultimately an overall increase in your pain.

When in bed, lie on your side and bend at your hips and knees to ninety degrees. Place a small pillow between your knees OR lie on your back with legs elevated by pillows. In this position your hips and knees are bent and the stress and pressure on your spine is at a minimum.

Ice and heat can relieve your back pain but you should understand how and why they work.

Ice reduces inflammation initially due to decreasing blood flow from constricted blood vessels and provides pain relief.

Heat causes blood vessels to expand, allowing more blood to flow to the affected area, thereby encouraging healing.

Method of ice application - Use a kitchen towel and apply ice pack on the towel over the affected area for up to twenty minutes every two hours.

Method of heat application - Over the years, I've seen different products claiming miracle results but the one method that has worked the most is wrapping a hot water bottle in a moist towel and placing on the affected area for twenty minutes every two hours. Sometimes the simplest approach works the best.

Which and when to apply:

Apply ice in the first forty-eight hours after the injury and then heat thereafter. The rationale behind this theory is that the ice helps reduce inflammation and provides more pain relief. After the initial swelling decreases, applying heat can help healing by causing more blood flow to the area.

Try anti-inflammatory drugs. Any over-the-counter anti-inflammatory medication can help decrease inflammation associated with your back pain and can provide some pain relief. Take your medicine according to the directions. Do not stop the medication because you feel slightly better. Taking medication at regular intervals, according to the directions, for about one or two weeks builds a level of medication in your blood that can continue to fight inflammation and provide pain relief over the course of your acute back pain flare-up.

Do not believe that 'more must be better'. Taking more medication than is recommended can have serious side-effects such as liver and kidney damage, among other things. One of the most common side effects of anti-inflammatory medications includes stomach upset, abnormal bleeding and ulcers. If you have problems with your stomach or gastrointestinal system you should check with your doctor before taking any of these medicines.

If your back pain does not improve after taking these medications for one or two weeks consult your doctor.

If you are on other medications for different medical problems, or if you have a medical problem in addition to your back pain, you should always consult with your doctor before self-medicating.

MOVE AROUND.

After a few days of bed rest, you should start gradually increasing your activity and overall time out of bed. Walking is an excellent exercise that is safe for your back and gets your blood flowing and stretches out your stiff muscles. Begin by walking around the inside of the house and progress to walking outside on a smooth flat even surface. Adjust your speed depending on your back pain, starting out very slowly and eventually working your way up to speed walking.

If walking is too much initially, try walking in a swimming pool. Walk across the shallow end. This exercise is easier on your body because it is almost weightless in water. You are placing minimal stress on your back and the water prevents you from doing any jerky or rapid movements. If your walking is going relatively well, you can add the back exercises discussed later.

CHAPTER 3:

- ## Common Medical Tests
- ## Invasive & Conservative Treatments
- ## When Surgery Is Necessary
- ## Different Types of Spine Surgery

Common Medical Tests:

Your doctor or health care professional gains the most important information from the history of your back pain problem and a physical examination. The most important diagnostic tool is a complete and thorough medical history.

The history should include at least the following factors:

How your back pain started: Did you have an accident or did you just wake up with the pain one day?

The course of your symptoms: Are your symptoms getting better or worse from the time you first noticed them? Are you experiencing any new symptoms? Have any symptoms come and gone?

Your current symptoms: Mention all the symptoms you currently experience (not only the pain, but also any weakness, sleep problems, depression).

A thorough physical examination helps determine whether you have any type of disc problem in your lower spine and where - at which level of the spine the problem has occurred. This includes looking at how you walk, stand and sit. Also palpating areas of your body where you complain of pain.

Straight leg test (sciatic nerve stretch test)

In this test, you lie flat on your back with your legs and feet extended fully on the exam table. The doctor then lifts one leg at a time to see whether doing so causes pain anywhere in either leg.

This test increases the tension in the nerve that goes from your back down your legs (sciatic nerve). If this test causes pain, it can be an indication as to whether you have an irritated nerve root.

Muscle Strength test:

Individual muscle groups of your lower body correspond to a specific nerve root level (the part of your lower spine, where the nerve exits the spine). If a nerve is injured, then the muscles that it controls may show weakness because your muscles are controlled by nerves. Strength tests are conducted to make sure that a nerve problem is not causing muscle weakness.

Many people are very quick and willing to accept that sophisticated machines such as MRI and CT scan are more accurate and more 'scientific'. However this is not always the case.

Sophisticated diagnostic tests, such as the MRI and CT scan are very sensitive and enable normal wear-and-tear changes in your spine be detected that couldn't be otherwise. Unfortunately, many specialists interpret these normal changes as 'abnormal' and proceed with inappropriate recommendations and treatments.

Before undergoing one of these tests ask the following questions:

- What is the test and what does it show?
- Why do you advise I have this test?
- What can I expect before, during and after the test?
- What does it mean if the test is positive or negative?
- Will the results of this test change my treatment plan? If not, then why put myself through the test?

THE DIAGNOSTIC TESTS:

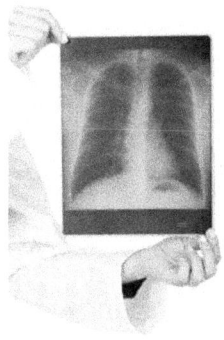

Plain X rays

An x-ray machine passes low-level radiation through part of your body, projecting a picture on a piece of film. The level of radiation from an X ray is very small. An X ray can show whether you are experiencing changes associated with normal ageing, fractures, and overall alignment of your spine.

<u>You may be an appropriate candidate for an X ray if</u>:

- You still have back pain after two or three weeks of conservative treatment.
- You have back pain even during periods of no activity
- You have back pain that awakens you from sleep at night
- You have back pain after a trauma or a fall

Supposedly 'abnormal' findings on your X ray, such as wear-and-tear changes that occur with ageing usually are not significant. In many cases they do not relate to the back pain that you are experiencing. Findings that may relate to your back pain include such conditions as a fracture, severe degeneration, or significant scoliosis.

Just because your X rays do not show anything significant does not mean that your pain is not real. The majority of painful back conditions probably come from the soft tissues of your spine including the muscles, tendons, discs and ligaments. X-rays see right through these.

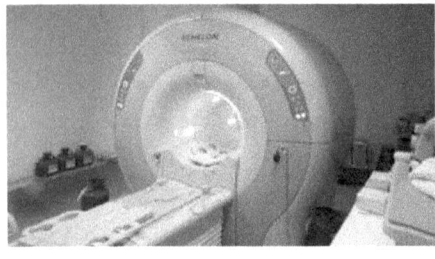

Magnetic Resonance Imaging (MRI).

The MRI shows nerves, muscles, ligaments and discs as well as the bones of the spine. This test gives much more information than X rays without exposing you to radiation.

An MRI may be appropriate for you if:

- You are a possible surgical candidate
- You still have back pain after six to eight weeks of appropriate, conservative treatment.
- There is a suspicion your pain may be related to an infection or tumor. (Severe pain that awakens you from sleep is often a symptom of infections and tumors).

The MRI test is extremely sensitive and can detect subtle changes in your spine that occur naturally as you age. These changes occur in people without back pain too especially if you are over thirty-five. The MRI procedure is safe and has almost no side effects. MRIs require no special preparation (e.g. fasting etc.). You lie down on a scanning table that slides into a giant magnet shaped like a large tube. Inside the tube, you hear several noises, including a humming sound and a thumping as the radio waves are turned on and off. The most difficult part of the test is lying still.

In some cases, you may undergo an MRI with a contrast agent, which is a fluid that is injected into your arm or leg prior to the test. This non-harmful substance can help provide an MRI picture that is much clearer, especially if you have had prior spine surgery. The contrast agent can help distinguish scar tissue, which may occur with prior surgery. If your doctor does not mention the possibility of using a contrast agent, ask - especially if you have had prior spine surgery.

An MRI cannot show some causes of pain such as a sprain-strain in the muscles or ligaments and stress- related back pain. Therefore, you can have normal test results and still have pain.

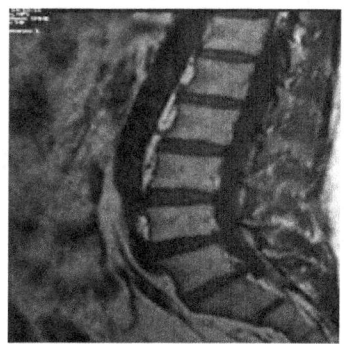

The CT scan
CT stands for computerized tomography also called a CAT scan, which is computerized axial tomography. A CT scan is a computerized recording of a slice or section of your body. The CT scan does not show your soft tissues, nerves and muscles quite as well as the MRI, but it does show the anatomy of the bony structures of your spine, as well as your discs and nerves.

41

<u>Your doctor may choose a CT scan for you over an MRI scan if</u>:

- You are very claustrophobic and can't tolerate being in the MRI machine even with a sedative.
- Your doctor needs to see the anatomy of your bony structures where the nerves exit the spinal canal.

The CT scan is also a cylinder-shaped machine, just like the MRI. You lie on your back for about thirty to forty-five minutes. Unlike the MRI, the tube is much larger and less likely to make you feel closed in if you are prone to claustrophobia. The test is painless. As with the MRI, in some cases you may have a CT scan with a contrast agent to help make certain aspects of the picture more visible.

ELECTRODIAGNOSTIC STUDIES

Electromyography (EMG) and nerve conduction studies (NCS) are the most common electro diagnostic studies - they are tests that measure the electrical activity and function of your nerves and muscles that your specialist may use in assessing your back pain.

The tests can show whether the electrical activity of various nerves has been disrupted. During the study, small needles are inserted into several of the muscles that are being assessed. In an EMG, these needles are connected to a monitor that shows the electrical activity of your nerves and muscles.

In a nerve conduction study, an electrical pulse stimulates ('*buzzes*') your nerves so that special receiving electrodes can monitor the electrical activity. You may experience mild to moderate pain with this test.

These tests can help determine a variety of diagnoses that involve problems with the nervous system or assess the re-growth of nerves after lumbar disc surgery for sciatica.

INVASIVE CONSERVATIVE TREATMENTS

Invasive conservative treatments are those in which your doctor actually pierces your skin as part of the treatment. These treatments are still considered 'conservative' because they are reversible. These treatments are usually reserved for those patients whose back pain problems do not respond to the non-invasive conservative treatments.

Trigger point injections:

A trigger point injection involves injecting a small amount of anaesthetic into certain muscle points or trigger points. Your doctor may give you trigger point injections if you seem to have areas of muscle that refer 'trigger' pain throughout a region of your body such as your lower or mid-back. For instance you may be able to point to certain specific areas in your back that, when pushed with your finger, seem to cause pain not only in that local area but also throughout an entire region of your back.

Facet injections

If your consultant thinks that your pain is coming from your facet joints, they may recommend facet injections. These injections use steroid or anesthetic to decrease the inflammation of the facet joint and provide pain relief.

Spinal epidural steroid injections.

In a spinal epidural steroid injection, your consultant uses a needle to inject steroid and sometimes an anesthetic into a specific area of your spinal canal. The consultant injects the steroid, which helps decrease inflammation and pain, into an area (or epidural space) that contains the disc and spinal nerves.

Your doctor may recommend epidural injections if some type of disc or nerve root irritation problem are contributing to your back pain and leg pain. Epidural injections are often done in series of three. Most consultants will not give you more than three epidural injections per six month period because too much steroid in your spine is not a good thing.

 Whether you will have more than one epidural injection really depends on your response to the first and the amount of steroid used. Recent research suggests that the full benefits of an epidural injection may not occur for a period of seven to ten days.

Selective nerve root blocks:

Selective nerve root blocks are similar to spinal epidural steroid injections but are directed more specifically to the exact source of your pain. They can be more effective than spinal epidural steroid injections in some cases. Steroids reduce inflammation of the disc or nerve root.

Rhizotomy

The purpose of a facet Rhizotomy injection is to provide lasting low back pain relief by disabling the sensory nerve that goes to the facet joint. In this injection procedure a needle with a probe is inserted just outside the joint. The probe is then heated with radio waves and applied to the sensory nerve to the joint in order to disable the nerve. Theoretically, by deadening the sensory nerve to the facet joint, a facet rhizotomy effectively prevents the pain signals from getting to the brain.

A facet rhizotomy injection is successful in providing lasting pain relief for approximately fifty percent of patients.

Surgery

Your doctor may suggest spine surgery in several situations:

- You have a certain condition (such as a spinal tumour or other emergency) that makes surgery medically necessary.

- You've completed a course of conservative treatment without getting better.

- The correlation between your symptoms and what appears to be causing your pain is high.

Spine surgery is elective in virtually all cases except emergency situations such as cauda equina syndrome, tumors, progressive neurological deficits, and some infections.

Cauda equina syndrome : In this extremely rare condition, important nerve roots in your lower spine, critical to bowel and bladder function and responsible for sensation to the groin and anal areas, are compressed (usually due to a herniated disc).

Symptoms of cauda equina syndrome include numbness in the genital region, around the anus, and in your feet; an inability to urinate; and the loss of sexual function. Without quick surgical treatment you may end up with permanent loss of bowel, bladder and sexual function.

Tumours: Surgery is frequently necessary to remove a spinal tumour. Even though a tumor may be non-cancerous and slow-growing, it can press on important parts of your spine, especially if the tumor is in your neck or mid-back area. A spine tumor may produce pain that awakens you from sleep, and/or you may be more comfortable sleeping in an upright position.

If your tumor is slow-growing, non-cancerous, and not pressing on any important spinal areas, you may not need surgery.

Infections: Just like any other part of your body, you can get an infection in your spine. Pain from a spinal infection is an intense, throbbing, aching kind of pain. It is often present at rest and awakens you from sleep.

Diagnosing a spinal infection can include the use of imaging tests, bone scans, and blood test. Doctors treat these infections with intravenous antibiotics. Some patient may need surgical treatment to clean out the infected area in addition to the antibiotics.

Questions to ask your consultant prior to surgery.

- What is my diagnosis and what does it mean for me?
- What is the natural pattern of my problem if left untreated?
- What are my treatment options?
- What are the risks and benefits of these options?
- Why are you recommending this specific course of treatment?
- What does the surgery entail?
- What are the possible complications and how do you treat them?
- How will I feel after surgery?
- How long will I be in the hospital?
- What will my recovery and rehabilitation be like?
- What preparations should I make to ensure that the surgery is as successful as possible?

Remember, in virtually all cases, you should get a second opinion regarding a proposed spine surgery. You only have one spine. Do not consider spine surgery without first thoroughly investigating non-surgical treatment options. You may be drawn to the quick-fix appeal of surgery but there is no guarantee that surgery will take care of your pain better than a conservative approach and the natural course of healing.

TYPES OF SURGERY

Lumbar decompression surgery is a type of spinal surgery. It is used to treat some types of back and leg pain, which have failed to respond to other treatments.

Decompression surgery is most commonly used to treat a condition called spinal stenosis. This is when a section of the spinal column becomes narrowed and places pressure on the nerves inside, leading to persistent pain and numbness and weakness in the lower back, buttocks and legs.

Decompression surgery can also be used to:

- Treat a slipped disc – where one of the discs becomes damaged and in some cases presses down on an underlying nerve

- Treat a spinal injury

- Relieve pressure on the spinal cord that is caused by an abnormal growth of tissue (tumour) – spinal tumours can be both cancerous and non-cancerous

- Relieve pressure on the spinal cord caused by cancer spreading into the spine – this is known as metastatic spinal cord compression

What happens during spinal surgery?

There are three main techniques used during spinal surgery:

Laminectomy – where a section of vertebrae (the lamina) is removed to relieve pressure on the affected nerve

Discectomy – where a section of a damaged disc is removed or destroyed to relieve pressure on a nerve

Spinal fusion – where two or more vertebrae are jointed together with a section of bone to strengthen the spine

In many cases, a combination of these techniques may be used.

For example, the surgeon may perform:

A laminectomy to gain better access to a damaged disc
Then a discectomy to remove a section of the disc
And then finally spinal fusion to reduce the chance of the spine becoming damaged again in the future.

Recovering from lumbar decompression surgery

Depending on the complexity of the surgery, you may be well enough to leave hospital one to ten days later.

You will need to avoid strenuous activities for around six weeks. Most people can return to work after this time.

Complications

An infection at the site of the incision is the most common complication of lumbar decompression surgery and will need to be treated with antibiotics. Post-operative infection occurs in approximately one in twenty-five cases.

More serious complications are rare and include:

Damage to the spinal cord resulting in some degree of paralysis (inability to move one or more parts of the body) – this is thought to occur in around one in three hundred cases

Death due to an unforeseen complication, such as a blood clot – this is thought to occur in around one in three hundred and fifty cases where surgery is used to treat spinal stenosis and one in seven hundred cases where surgery is used to treat a slipped disk

CHAPTER 4:

<u>Complementary Approaches</u>

- **Acupuncture**
- **Pilates**
- **Yoga**

Many people suffering from a variety of health problems (including back pain) look toward alternative medicine approaches for relief. It is the author's experience that the most powerful approach is the combination of the two orientations in an appropriate manner.

<u>The following guidelines are to assist you in seeking out an expert in complementary medicine:</u>

Find a practitioner with whom you can establish a good rapport. As with any doctor, you want to find a complementary medicine practitioner with whom you feel comfortable. A good relationship with your health practitioner includes such elements as open communication and an overall sense of trust in that person's abilities.

<u>Rely on a referral source that you trust:</u>

One of the best (and most common) ways to find a good practitioner is through a referral, either from your doctor or from someone who has been treated by the individual. Talking to someone who has been treated by the practitioner can give you a good idea about that person's bedside manner, conduct and practices.

Select a practitioner who is sensitive to your needs: Find a practitioner who has experience treating back pain.

Beware of a practitioner who is not willing to work with your doctor. Successful treatment of conditions such as chronic back pain is often a collaborative effort by a variety of different healthcare professionals. If any practitioner is unwilling to work with other disciplines you have found helpful, this refusal can be a warning sign of a problem.

Beware of quick fixes:

Quacks can often claim that their treatments or remedies can produce immediate cures. If you have chronic back pain, you may be more susceptible to claims for a quick fix due to your frustration over the ongoing pain and desire for relief.

If your problem has been going on for over three months, the improvement usually begins slowly and gradual. In addition, regardless of the chosen therapy, you may not see improvement in all of your symptoms simultaneously. It is always a good idea to keep in mind the 'three steps forward, one step back' rule. In treatment of back pain problems, one has often seen patients move forward in terms of feeling better and becoming more active, only to have an occasional set-back. Remember, if you move three steps forward and one step backward in your treatment, you are still two steps ahead. Keeping this rule in mind prevents you from getting discouraged when set-backs or flare-ups occur.

Remember no one (including your doctor) knows exactly how long effective treatment will take. On average uncomplicated cases should take less than eight weeks. You should try eight - twelve sessions and stopping if there is no lasting improvement at that point.

Factors that may make recovery take longer include:

- Symptoms that have been present longer than eight days
- Severe symptoms that are not getting better on their own
- A history of more than three prior episodes of the same problem
- Presence of another problem in your bones or joints (arthritis, disc degeneration or herniation)

COMPLEMENTARY THERAPIES

ACUPUNCTURE

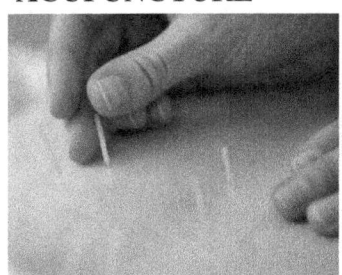

What is acupuncture?

Acupuncture is a treatment that consists in pricking the patient with a special needle. It developed in China about 2,000 years ago. Traditional Chinese acupuncture uses a complicated system of ancient ideas that are not easy for most of us to understand or accept today.

However, many modern Western practitioners find that acupuncture can be understood in scientific terms. This makes it easier to use in a Western setting and it is becoming increasingly acceptable here. Many hospitals today offer acupuncture to their patients and the British Medical Acupuncture Society has over 2500 members.

Today, therefore, there are two main forms of acupuncture: traditional and modern.

The differences are mainly at the level of theory - ideas about what is going on when one inserts an acupuncture needle into a patient. There, are, however, also some practical differences.

Modern acupuncturists do not use traditional diagnostic methods such as the pulse or the appearance of the tongue.

Many, though not all, modern acupuncturists leave the needles in place for quite a short time: often about two minutes or even less.

Many, though not all, modern acupuncturists use only a few needles - perhaps four and sometimes only one.

Surprising though this may seem, experience shows that doing acupuncture this way is as effective as using a lot of needles and leaving them in for longer and is less likely to have unwanted effects.

Which is better, modern or traditional?

It is not possible to give an objective answer to this question because there is little good research evidence that bears on it. Probably both versions of acupuncture are roughly similar in effectiveness but modern acupuncture is generally quicker and easier to perform. There are also some techniques in the modern version that are not used in traditional acupuncture and which are particularly effective in certain circumstances, e.g. for the treatment of joint pain (arthritis).

How does it work?

In many cases the acupuncturist makes use of "trigger points". These are areas, usually in muscle, that hurt when pressed and cause pain to radiate to other places that may be some distance away from the trigger point. Needling the trigger point can relieve pain in these distant areas, although we do not know exactly how this happens.

Acupuncture can still work even when there are no trigger points. In such cases it probably acts by changing the ways in which the central nervous system (brain and spinal cord) is transmitting information about pain.

It is important to understand that acupuncture does have measurable effects on the body even though we can't explain them all in detail. You do not have to believe in it for it to work!

What diseases can be helped by acupuncture?

It is not possible to give a complete list, partly because a lot depends on the reaction of the individual patient.

Some people are much better subjects than others, and some do not respond at all.

In general, acupuncture is good for pain, especially pain in the muscles and joints (including some kinds of arthritis). It can also help in a range of other disorders, including headaches and migraine, some allergies, painful periods, and ulcerative colitis.

Does it hurt?

Acupuncture is usually not pain-free. However, it is no more painful than an ordinary injection or blood test and in many cases it is less painful than these. As a rule it is necessary to produce a little pain to achieve an improvement but some people feel nothing at all. Oddly enough, you may even find that acupuncture makes you feel relaxed and happy. If this happens it probably means that you are a good acupuncture subject and are likely to benefit from this form of treatment. (If it does not happen to you, however, that is not a bad sign; you may do well anyway.)

Can it cause any harm?

Acupuncture carries the same risks as any other medical procedure involving needles, such as damage to internal organs or structures, though this is rare. To put it in perspective, the risk of harm occurring as the result of acupuncture is probably less than the risk of taking aspirin or an anti-inflammatory drug for arthritis (these drugs can cause bleeding). This assumes, of course, that the acupuncture is performed by someone with an adequate knowledge of anatomy and medicine.

Are there any particular adverse effects I should look out for?

Sometimes a small bruise appears where the needle was inserted. This is not serious; it just means that a little vein was broken by the needle. There is no need to do anything about it; it will go away by itself.

Some patients find that their symptoms become temporarily worse for a short time after acupuncture. This is termed an aggravation. Tell the person who is treating you about this next time you come; it may be possible to avoid the aggravation in future by treating you more lightly, with fewer needles or for a shorter time. But some people will get a mild aggravation every time they have acupuncture. In general, aggravation is followed by an improvement, so it is quite a good sign.

Some degree of drowsiness after acupuncture is fairly common. This may make driving or operating machinery dangerous, so patients should generally not drive themselves home after treatment, particularly on the first occasion. Sometimes drowsiness does not occur after the first treatment but does occur on a subsequent occasion, and it is also possible for the onset of drowsiness to occur later in the day, some hours after treatment. Patients who have had acupuncture should therefore be cautious about driving for the rest of the day and should be prepared for their reflexes to be slower than normal.

This list does not exhaust all the adverse effects that have been reported but it does summarize the commonest ones. If you have any particular anxieties about the treatment you should discuss them with the person who is going to treat you.

Can acupuncture transmit Aids or hepatitis?

No, because all the needles are disposed of after use. There is therefore no possibility that infection could be transmitted.

How soon will I notice an improvement?

Some patients notice partial or even complete relief as soon as the needle is put in but this is exceptional. Most find that improvement takes longer to appear - sometimes later the same day or perhaps up to two or three days.

How many treatments will I require?

Sometimes one treatment is enough but this is unusual. Most people require a course of roughly three to six treatments. At first you may be asked to come back after one or two weeks; as improvement occurs the intervals between treatments may be made longer.

Generally speaking, there should be at least some effect after two or three treatments. If nothing at all happens you are probably not going to respond to this form of treatment.

You may find that the effects of treatment vary from time to time. One treatment may help a lot, the next less or even not at all. Do not worry too much about this; provided there is a long-term trend towards improvement all is in order.

Will acupuncture cure me completely?

This depends on what you are being treated for. Some illnesses can be cured, and many more can be helped a lot although not completely cured. In such cases you may need to have repeated treatments at intervals, perhaps once every two or three months.

PILATES

Pilates is a system of physical conditioning developed by Joseph Pilates almost a century ago. It has a strong emphasis on proper body alignment, injury prevention, and correct breathing, as well as muscle stretching and strengthening.

Pilates is appropriate for people of all ages, abilities and lifestyles, including those suffering from back pain.

Pilates emphasizes muscle stretching and its goal is to promote muscle elongation, rather than building bulk. Pilates attempts to develop your abdomen and lower back into a firm core of support for your whole body. The program promotes alignment, balance and stabilization of your spine which, in turn, makes it easier to work other parts of your body.

Therapeutic Massage:

Massage is one of the most frequently used therapies for musculoskeletal problems, particularly for controlling pain. Research indicates that therapeutic massage can have several beneficial effects on low back pain including:

- Relaxing the nervous system and muscles
- Breaking down scar tissue and lessening fibrosis and adhesions that develop as a result of injury
- Helping to reduce swelling
- Improving blood flow through the muscles.

Therapeutic massage releases muscle tension and promotes relaxation. Muscle tension (either from activity, injury or stress) may contribute to muscle fatigue and pain by pushing on nerve fibres in the muscle.

Muscle contraction (tightening) for an extended period of time interferes with the elimination of chemical waste products in the muscles and surrounding tissues.

The longer a muscle is tense, the more these chemical waste products build up and irritate the nerves and muscles in the area, causing more pain. Therapeutic massage can help break up these muscular waste deposits and stimulate more blood flow to the painful areas.

YOGA

Yoga is one of the oldest known systems of health practice in the world. The breathing exercises, physical postures and mediation practices of yoga can help you with reducing stress, regulating heart rate, lowering blood pressure and relieving pain.

One of the common causes of back problems may be prolonged over- stretching of the back ligaments and muscles due to poor posture during sitting and standing, but probably mostly sitting. Most people bend forward too much throughout the day. Poor posture takes a toll on your body - especially your back - after days, weeks and years of repetition causing chronic physical problems

Yoga therapy can be an excellent approach either by itself or as part of an overall treatment plan for your back problem.

CHAPTER 5: POWER OF THE MIND

When subjected to the same painful stimulus, different individuals may experience differing levels of intensity and unpleasantness. In addition, one individual may feel different levels of pain depending on the situation.

Thus, the nervous system and the brain are not a purely reactive stimulus/response machine when it comes to pain. There are steps in between the sensation and perception (a cognitive interpretation of the sensations) that determine how the pain is experienced.

Some researchers claim that in order to feel pain, one needs to attend to and process the stimulus in an emotional way. If pain is not attended to or processed in a certain way then it might not reach the level of conscious awareness. Thus, how much attention one gives to pain determines how intense and unpleasant the sensation will be.

There are many situations in which an individual might not attend to their pain as much as they normally would—such as a stressful situation like war or in competitive situations like a sports event. There are countless stories of athletes and soldiers being terribly injured and only realizing after the event that something was wrong.

Normally, pain serves to notify us of a problem and point our attention towards it. This way we can alter our behavior in such a way that we can treat the injury and somehow reduce the pain. But there are times when we have bigger problems than pain— such as survival, when attending to an injury could be costly or even fatal. (For instance, in our evolutionary past, if we were injured and being chased by a tiger.)

There is scientific evidence that individuals in much less stressful settings can be distracted in various ways so that they do not feel as much pain. And likewise, paying attention to a painful stimulus increases its intensity ratings.

We all have a finite pool of attention that we must divide between different tasks or stimuli. Thus, if a good amount of attention is devoted to an activity, there is less attention available to devote to the processing of the pain.

Many factors - physical, mental, and emotional influence your back pain. You can have severe pain with minimal physical findings and minimal pain with horrendous findings. Your mind can influence your body in significant ways including whether you experience certain types of back pain, such as stress-related back pain.

Stress generally can be defined as a mental or physical demand made upon the body. Your body responds to stress by increasing your blood pressure and heart rate, causing rapid breathing, tensing your muscles, and reducing blood flow to your head, stomach, skin, hands, and feet.

When you are tense, your body also produces stress hormones to give you an energy burst. If you are in danger, these hormones help your body perform at maximum efficiency for survival reasons. But, when these hormones are released inappropriately over a long time, they damage your body. It is like running your car's engine beyond the design capabilities: It's okay for a quick get-away, but will blow up the engine if done extensively.

Scientific studies suggest that up to 85 percent of all medical problems are caused by stress. Prolonged stress causes physical changes in your body that result in various medical conditions. For example, stress-related problems can include such things as headaches, back pain, sleep problems, digestive disorders and high-blood pressure. Stress can make virtually any medical problem worse, and can make a surgical procedure more difficult at every stage.

Thoughts and emotions have a significant influence over our pain level and suffering. We constantly evaluate the world around us. We constantly evaluate the sensations going on inside our body as well. These constant thoughts are automatic thoughts because they occur almost automatically, outside of our awareness.

Automatic thoughts tend to be very fast, unconscious, and highly credible. Automatic thoughts have huge influence over your emotions, behaviours and pain. Research shows that human beings under stress have a tendency to engage in irrational negative automatic thoughts.

Negative automatic thoughts tend to produce negative emotions such as depression, anxiety and fear as well as increased pain sensations.

Experiencing back pain is often a stressful situation - one that can result in a variety of negative automatic thoughts, including some of the following:

- I will never get better.
- My back is getting worse and worse
- I am going to end up a cripple
- Why is this happening to me?

Most of my patients acknowledge having the preceding types of thoughts at one time or another. Coping or rational, thoughts are directly opposed to negative automatic thoughts. Coping thoughts reflect the true reality of the situation and help you focus on the range of options available to help solve a problem like back pain.

<u>Coping thoughts may be similar to the following</u>:

- Because no one can predict the future, I benefit more by being optimistic than pessimistic.

- This pain does not mean that I am getting worse, I am showing improvement in the following ways

- I have no evidence that this back pain is going to make me a cripple.

- I am going to think about what I can do to better my situation instead of spending my time asking why this happened to me.

You do not have to be a victim of negative automatic thoughts. You can learn how to identify negative automatic thoughts as they occur and replace them with coping or nurturing thoughts. Remember negative thoughts can cause negative emotions such as depression, anxiety, fear, and anger which can in turn worsen your back pain. Then in a vicious cycle, the back pain causes more stress, resulting in a cascade of more negative automatic thoughts.

Relaxation Response:

It is important to distinguish between the 'relaxation response' and simply 'relaxing'. The relaxation response involves a number of physical changes, including:

- Decrease in heart rate
- Decrease in respiration rate
- Decrease in blood pressure
- Decrease in muscle tension
- Decrease in metabolism rate and oxygen consumption.

Practice once or twice a day. Practicing at least once a day is necessary in order to elicit the relaxation response. Initially your relaxation sessions may take more time. As you practice regularly, you may find that the amount of time required to elicit the relaxation response decreases.

- Find a quiet location.

- Practice your exercises in a location where you will not be disturbed or distracted.

- Turn off your phone, use a fan or meditation music to block out outside noise while you are practicing.

- Give a five-minute warning. Give yourself and other family members a five-minute warning before you begin your exercises.

- Practice at regular times. Setting up regular practice times increases the likelihood that you will follow through on your relaxation exercises. Choose a time when you are most likely to follow through on completing the exercises. Your regular practice times should not be when you are so tired that you are likely to fall asleep (right after a big meal or just prior to bed)

- Assume a comfortable position. A common position is lying flat on your back with legs extended and your arms comfortably at your sides. Depending upon your back pain, you may want to flex your knees, or support them with a pillow. If this position still causes pain, you can complete relaxation exercises while sitting or standing.

- Loosen your clothing: Loosen any tight clothing and take off such things as shoes, belt, watch, glasses, and jewelry. The objective is to be as comfortable as possible while you practice the exercises. Try writing down all the things on your mind, and then physically putting the paper aside prior to practicing. You can focus better on the relaxation exercise if your other concerns are documented for your attentions AFTER you finish.

- Assume a passive attitude. You need to allow the relaxation response to happen. You should not try to relax or control your body. Focusing on your breathing is all you need to do. Relaxation occurs on its own.

Achieving the relaxation response reduces generalized anxiety, prevents stress from building up over time, increases energy levels and productivity, and improves concentration, memory and ability to focus. It induces deeper, more restorative sleep and a reduction of insomnia and fatigue. It increases awareness of your actual emotional state and feelings. The following is an example of a breathing exercise that is an excellent method of inducing the relaxation response.

Lying down as described earlier or sitting upright, take three complete breaths focusing on breathing from your diaphragm.

To do this follow the next steps.

Close your eyes and place one hand on your breastbone and the other hand over your belly button.

Without trying to change how you normally breathe, become aware of which part of your body is moving as you inhale and exhale. The hand on you breastbone monitors chest breathing, and the hand over your belly button monitors abdominal breathing.

Pay attention to which hand rises when you inhale - the one on your abdomen or the one on your chest. If your abdomen moves up and down with each breath, you are breathing diaphragmatically. If your abdomen does not move up and down then you need to practice the following steps.

Gently place both of your hands (or a book) on your abdomen (bellybutton) and again focus on your breathing. Pay attention to how your abdomen rises as you inhale and falls as you exhale. Try to make your hands rise and fall as you inhale and exhale - rise when you inhale, fall when you exhale. Breathe through your nose during this exercise. Press your hand down on your abdomen as you exhale (breathe out) and allow your abdomen to push your hand back up as you inhale (breathe in) deeply.

The pressure from your hand helps you become more aware of the action of your abdomen during breathing. You are inhaling and exhaling should be of equal length as well as being slow, controlled, and smooth.

After taking the three complete breaths, complete the following.

Close your right nostril with the thumb of your right hand and breathe out completely through your left nostril.

After you have exhaled completely, close your left nostril with your right index finger and inhale completely through your right nostril.

Repeat this cycle of breathing out through your left nostril and inhaling through your right nostril two more times. Be sure that you maintain an equal length of time for inhaling and exhaling.

At the end of inhaling the third time through the right nostril, exhale completely through the SAME (right) nostril, while keeping the left nostril closed. At the end of this exhalation, close your right nostril and inhale through your left nostril.

Repeat this cycle of exhaling through your right nostril and inhaling through your left nostril two more times.

Then place your hands on your knees while exhaling and inhaling through both nostrils evenly for three complete breaths.

The following is a summary of the entire exercise:

- Complete breaths, both nostrils Three times
- Exhale left and inhale right Three times
- Exhale right and inhale left Three times
- Complete breaths, both nostrils Three times.

CHAPTER 6: Common Questions about Back Pain

1. Can I Manage My Herniated Disc without Surgery?
2. Why Do I Still Have Pain When My Imaging Scans Are Normal?
3. Is My Diagnosis as Terrible as It Sounds?
4. When Should I Consider Surgery for My Back Pain Problem?
5. Can Stress and Emotions Cause My Back Pain?
6. How Can Pain Only in My Legs Be Related to My Back?
7. Should I Continue Exercising if doing so worsens my pain and what about a back support?
8. What about Sex?

Over the years, questions and worries that people suffering from back pain have repeat themselves with remarkable frequency. This chapter is dedicated to those people and their questions.

1. Can I Manage My Herniated Disc

You can almost always manage your herniated disc successfully without surgery. Only a very small percentage of patients actually require surgery. Many research studies show that patients with a herniated disc can recover well with non-surgical conservative management. In one study, ninety-two per cent of patients with documented disc herniation recovered without surgery. * *J.A. Saal et al 'The Natural History of Lumbar Intervertebral Disc Extrusions Treated Non-operatively' Spine 15 (1990): 8-20).*

Many of these patients had large herniated discs that were compressing nerve roots. In another study, patients with disc herniation were treated either surgically or non-surgically. After five years, the researchers found no difference in the groups. * *H. Weber, 'Lumbar Disc Herniation: A controlled, Prospective Study with Ten years of Observation' Spine 8 1983 131-140).*

One often sees symptoms of a herniated disc with nerve compression (back pain, buttock pain, and sciatica) resolve spontaneously as the disc shrinks. Your body has a natural ability to heal and reabsorb disc herniation and return to a normal state.

Surgery may be appropriate for your disc herniation in some cases. If your neurological symptoms, such as weakness in your legs, decreased sensation, and bowel and/or bladder problems, are getting progressively worse, your doctor may recommend surgery to prevent permanent neurological damage.

2. Why do I still have Pain when my Imaging scans are normal?

Many known and well-understood structural reasons for back pain may be applicable to your specific problem. However, in a large percent of all back pain cases, doctors find no specific, identifiable structural diagnosis. One reason your scans may be normal while you still have discomfort is that your back pain may come from sources that current imaging technology cannot identify. In fact, high-tech instruments may never be able to identify things like pain from inflammation, sprain or strain in the muscles or ligaments, and back pain due to unconscious mental stress.

Imaging studies are not the definitive answer to diagnosing back pain. The results can be difficult to interpret because people with no back pain can have abnormal MRIs while people with back pain often have normal MRIs. Imaging studies and high-tech assessments are only one part of a good back pain evaluation.

The prognosis for a full recovery is extremely good even if your doctors never find the exact cause of your back pain. Treatments often work whether you know the exact cause of pain or not.

3. Is My Diagnosis as terrible as it sounds?

Doctors may use a number of scary sounding spinal diagnoses even though the reality of the condition may be nothing serious at all. Two such examples are disc protrusion or bulge and degenerative disc disease. Many diagnoses were not at all common prior to the event of sophisticated imaging studies such as MRI and CT scan. Unfortunately, practitioners often over-interpret these imaging studies as being abnormal rather than as simply a part of normal wear-and-tear changes in the spine as you age.

Disc bulges are not a cause for concern and in fact, are present in a high percentage of the population who do not have any back pain or symptoms. Similarly, so-called arthritis of the spine and degenerative changes are most often not associated with any back symptoms. Spinal degeneration actually starts when you are about twenty years of age and continues throughout your lifetime. In the vast majority of cases, you should think of this condition as similar to other ageing processes, such as your hair turning gray.

4. When Should I Consider Surgery for my back pain problem?

Surgery is medically necessary to correct only a few spinal problems. These conditions include severe nerve compression in the lower spine, spinal tumours, and some spinal infections. Consider surgery only after appropriate conservative treatment in most cases. Make sure that your surgeon has a very good idea of what is causing your pain and that surgery can correct the problems. Be sure that your objective findings - such as the physical examination and imaging studies closely match your subjective findings such as your complaints about the symptoms. Do not agree to exploratory surgery. Your surgeon should have a pretty good idea of what he or she is going to surgically correct. Make sure that you have no other issue that may ruin your response to surgery such as other medical problems. Get a second surgical opinion that is in agreement with the surgery recommendation before proceeding. Consider surgery only if your back pain is interfering with your quality of life to an unacceptable point.

5. Can Stress and Emotions Cause My Back Pain?

Thoughts and emotions are part of any back pain problem. Take this issue seriously if you believe - or your doctor suggests - that stress is making your back pain worse. Your brain evaluates all pain impulses and either amplifies or minimizes them. Your thoughts and emotions (and the resulting stress you experience) have great power over the way you perceive pain: Stress and emotions can worsen any pain impulses coming from your back.

Stress and emotions can actually cause your back pain. Although the exact mechanism is not clear, doctors think that unconscious stress causes muscle tightness in your lower back. The resulting pain is similar to having a tension or stress headache in your back. In this situation, your back pain originates entirely from emotional stress, and traditional medical treatments are not likely to be effective until you address the emotional stress.

Stress causes harmful effects on your body, including elevated blood pressure, elevated heart rate, increased muscle tension, rapid and shallow breathing, release of stress hormones, and reduced blood flow to certain areas of the body, diminished immune system function, and slower tissue-healing time.

6. How can pain only in my legs be related to my back?

Depending on the patient, this can be a difficult concept to explain. It is what is called referred pain. Perhaps the best way to describe this is by comparing your nerves to a telephone line.

Think of a telephone line extending from the telephone exchange terminal to your home. If the line just outside the exchange has a problem, you experience static on your telephone even though you may be several miles away.

Spinal nerves travel into your buttocks, down your legs, and all the way to your toes. If anything irritates those nerves, you can experience pain along the nerve. Thus, irritation of certain nerves in the lower spine can cause pain as far down as your feet and toes even if you do not experience any back pain, buttock pain, or upper leg pain.

7. Should I continue exercising if doing so worsens my pain and what about back supports?

In the acute or initial stages of your back pain problem, let pain be your guide. It's probably best to take two days of relative bed rest - up to five days only if necessary.

After acute onset of your back pain; then a gradual increase in your activities is recommended. As you increase your activities and add an exercise program at this stage, stop or reduce it if your pain worsens. Letting pain be your guide also applies to other spinal conditions that require a certain healing time such as a spinal fracture or recovery from a fusion surgery.

If a chronic back pain condition causes deconditioning (you become physically weak from not using your muscles) you can expect to experience an increase in pain with your exercise program. This increase in pain is similar to the aches and pains you experience after a good workout at the gym, because you are using muscles that you have not used for a while. In this case, you are experiencing 'good pain' because the pain indicates that you are getting stronger.

Even if you are receiving physical rehabilitation, you should still consult your doctor if exercise causes your back pain to worsen. Your doctor will make sure that the pain is part of the rehabilitation process and that you have no other problems or re-injuries.

Back braces/Supports: Many of my patients have heard that back supports cause muscle weakness and atrophy. This general belief is a myth. Lumbar supports can be worn daily without causing muscle weakness or atrophy as long as you continue to exercise your back muscles.

The final question that I am often asked –

8. <u>What about sex?</u>

This is a significant worry for a lot of back pain sufferers. Frustration, anger, guilt, fear and depression can all accompany a serious back problem. These emotions, along with the physical aspect of having back pain, can virtually wipe out any type of sexual relationship. Back pain can diminish your physical ability to have enjoyable intimacy as well as decrease your libido.

Back pain is invisible, which can cause even more problems in a couple's physical relationship. If you are the person in the relationship who is coping with back pain, you may begin to feel inadequate and experience self-critical thoughts such as 'Why would anybody want to be with me; I am an invalid'.

If your partner is dealing with back pain, your thoughts and emotions can also affect your physical relationship. You may be afraid that you may further injure your partner during any type of physical interaction. As a result, you do not initiate intimacy. If you withdraw from physical interaction, your partner may misinterpret these signals as having something to do with a lack of attraction on your part.

Many people have difficulty communicating openly about sex usually due to the attitude their parents left them with from childhood or cultural pressures that such talk is taboo. When couples cannot openly communicate about their sexual relationship, problems occur.

Physical intimacy can include activities that help you manage your back pain more effectively. Many individuals with back pain obtain relief from massage, hot packs, or taking a hot bath. You can incorporate all of these pain-relieving activities into your intimate activities. If back pain has had a very significant impact on your sexual relationship, you should begin slowly in terms of building sexual activity back into the relationship.

Open communication is vital. If your back pain is severe, take a more passive role in love-making initially. Talk to your partner about needing to be more passive at first until you work up to being able to tolerate greater activity. Discussing this issue openly will help you feel more comfortable about being passive and your partner will understand that you are not simply being selfish.

Getting Physical:

If you have back pain, you may find that lying on your back on a firm surface and placing your legs on pillows is a comfortable position. You may also gain comfort by rolling or folding a small hand towel under your lower back, giving it a slight arch and providing additional support for your back. This position is fairly passive for the person with back pain.

The missionary position is basically the man is on top and the woman is on the bottom.

<u>The missionary position can be fairly comfortable for a woman with back pain</u>:

Lie on your back with your legs bent, which allows you to maintain some curve in your spine. The degree your spine curves is relative to how close you bring your knees to your chest. If this position is not comfortable, try placing a towel or small pillow under your lower back to help keep it somewhat arched. You can then adjust how much you bend your legs.

By changing your position and lying on your stomach you can provide the most comfort for your back by placing a pillow under your chest or stomach, or propping yourself up on your elbows. If you have one-sided back pain problems, lie on your back with one knee bent up and the other leg lying flat.

<u>A man with back pain can benefit from the missionary position in the following ways</u>:

A modified missionary position can be particularly useful for one-sided back pain. Place a pillow or two underneath your partner to raise her buttocks. You can then lie between her legs with one of your legs bent into a deep kneeling position, keeping your other leg straight behind you. Which leg you bend and which leg you keep straight depends on which side you have back pain.

The female superior position:
The female superior position is simply woman on top. This position can be useful for both men and women with back pain.

For the man with back pain:
In the female superior position you can keep your back comfortable and non-stressed by straightening your knees or bending them more upwards, depending on what is most comfortable. You can also adjust your position by using towels and pillows for support. This passive position allows you to protect your back. Your partner's movements can range from very gentle to more physically active. Keep her informed of your comfort level, so she can adjust her movements in order to keep your pain at a minimum.

For the woman with back pain:
This position allows you virtually complete control over physical movement. You can control the depth of penetration and speed of thrust depending on your back pain. You can lay your chest down on your partner's which may be more comfortable if rounding out your back reduces pain. A variation on the standard female superior position is to face away from your partner. Try this variation to see whether it provides you with more comfort for your back.

Remember you won't know how it is going to affect your pain unless you try, and if at first it does not work, try a variation but communication is key and do not let fear rule you..

CHAPTER 7:
RED FLAGS AND ATTENDING YOUR DOCTOR

You can do a tremendous amount to manage your back pain at home, on your own but there are times when you need expert help.

There are a number of warning signs, known as 'red flags', which may indicate that your back pain is serious.

These red flag signs include:

- A high temperature (fever) of 38C (100F) or above
- Unexplained weight loss
- Constant back pain that does not ease after lying down or resting
- Pain that travels to your chest or that is high up in your back
- Pain down your legs and below the knees
- A recent trauma or injury to your back
- Loss of bladder control
- Inability to pass urine
- Loss of bowel control
- Numbness around your genitals, buttocks or back passage

If you have any of the signs or symptoms listed above, contact your GP immediately. You should also seek medical advice if you are having back pain and:

- You are under 20 or over 55 years old
- You have taken steroids for a few months
- You misuse drugs
- You have or have had cancer
- You have a weakened immune system as a result of chemotherapy treatment or a medical condition such as HIV or AIDS.
- Also contact your GP if your symptoms fail to improve within three days or you have persistent pain that lasts longer than six weeks.

Many of my patients often avoid going to the doctor, they give reasons such as
- My doctor does not spend enough time with me
- My doctor is not friendly
- All he does is write a prescription
- He never examines me
- My doctor does not explain problems understandably

The ability to work with your doctor and other treatment providers effectively is a critical part of enhancing your response to treatment. Your personal communication style can have a great impact on the doctor-patient relationship.

A suggestion when dealing with your doctor is to communicate in an assertive fashion. Assertive communication allows you to express how you feel or what you want while respecting the rights of others.

Use assertive nonverbal behaviour: Your body language goes beyond your verbal expression. Assertive behavior includes such things as establishing eye contact with your doctor, keeping your head up, standing straight, maintaining an open posture (facing your doctor with your head up and arms uncrossed), and staying calm. Your attitude about your doctor visit can affect the outcome greatly. If you are angry because you are in pain, you are likely to be aggressive. This does not lead to a pleasant and productive visit.

Whereas it is not productive to be aggressive, do not apologise for your request either. If you tend to be non-assertive, you may have trouble believing yourself that your request deserves a response. With an apologetic approach, your actual request is often ignored for example *'I am really sorry to ask, but could you, if possible, explain the test results again?'* replace this with a more assertive **'I would appreciate it if you would explain the test results again.'**

However at the same time remember do not make demands. Assertive communication involves either making a request of another person - not a demand or setting a limit by saying 'No.'. Always communicate in a way that respects the rights and dignity of the other person.

Allow your doctor to ask questions first. Your doctor needs to gather a great deal of information in a relatively short period of time, so let him or her ask questions first. After that, you can ask for any information not covered or that is unclear. Even though waiting to tell your doctor information what you think is important can be difficult, resist the urge to go into the visit with a prepared monologue because you may end up giving the doctor information that is not relevant to your diagnosis and treatment.

Your doctor will usually open with questions about how you are doing and what symptoms you are experiencing. This is your opportunity to tell your doctor what is going on. The doctor has to gather certain information in order to formulate a treatment plan and assess your progress. After he obtains that information, you can express your specific questions and concerns.

A common perception is that doctors do not value their patients' time but demand that patients honor theirs. Most doctors will keep their patients waiting only when uncontrollable circumstances arise (such as an urgent phone call related to patient care, an emergency patient visit or a consultation that goes on longer than expected). Unfortunately, these unforeseen problems causing delays happen more frequently than in other lines of work. Although you may feel as if you should be able to spend as much time with your doctor as you like (and ask as many questions as you want), this simply cannot happen. Your doctor needs to balance the time available for all patients throughout the day.

Planning your doctor visit in advance:

Before you see your doctor, think about what you want to get out of this particular visit and then make a list of your questions and concerns in a simple and straight forward format. You should be able to summarize them into about five main questions, which will allow adequate time for discussion.

Writing the questions down on a piece of paper and bringing them with you helps ensure that you get the information you require.

Communicating your goals at the outset can help the visit go smoothly.

Medical Fact Sheet:

Preparing a written summary of your important medical information can help you get the best possible treatment while avoiding any dangerous or harmful mistakes. Do not have the attitude *'he's my doctor, he should know'*. It is your health, your back and your responsibility. Preparing a medical fact sheet allows you to be an active participant in your treatment.

Your sheet should be concise and neat and include at least the following information:

- Your name, address, phone numbers, emergency contacts, and any special problems or disabilities.
- Current medical conditions with brief explanations
- Previous treatments and your response
- Previous tests (such as an MRI) and the results
- Past medical conditions with brief explanations and dates
- Surgical history with dates and outcomes
- Current medications with dosages and side effects
- Allergic reactions to medications.

Your Questions:

Keep your request simple. An assertive request is simple direct and straightforward. Ask for only one thing at a time, because a multitude of questions can be confusing for your doctor. Avoid vague requests and be specific regarding your wants, needs and feelings.

Bring a friend:

Bringing a friend or family member is an effective way to get the most out of your doctor visit- especially if you are facing an important medical decision. Your friend or family member's presence has a calming and relaxing effect, allowing you to focus better. You are less likely to feel intimidated with someone else along. Your companion can also bring up questions or concerns and help you recall the discussion with the doctor. If you and your companion do not agree on what was heard then you can raise these questions with your doctor on the next visit.

This now brings us to the second part of this chapter - the red flags or reasons when you must see your doctor and nobody else.

You are Weak in the Legs (or Feet)

If you begin to experience weakness in one or both of your legs and or feet, go to your doctor as quick as you can. With foot drop, your foot becomes so weak that you have trouble pulling your toes up toward your head, causing your foot to 'drop' and drag when you walk. Nerve compression in your spine may be the cause.

You Can't Control your bowels or bladder:

If you experience a loss of bowel or bladder control, see your doctor or go straight to the hospital. Also if you have any of the following:

- Loss of feeling during a bowel movement
- Inability to start or control your bowel movements
- Inability to start or control urination
- Loss of feeling to your groin or anal area

Cauda equina syndrome as mentioned in previous chapters may cause the preceding symptoms. The cauda equina syndrome involves a compression or 'pressing' on important nerves in your lower spine. These nerves supply function to your bowels and bladder, as well as sensation to your groin and anal areas. This condition usually requires quick, surgical treatment because permanent damage can occur if the nerves are compressed for too long.

Your Back Pain wakes you up:

If you have a back pain problem, pain may awaken you from sleep at night every once in a while. However, in some cases - rest pain that is back pain that consistently awakens you from sleep at night - can indicate a spinal infection or tumour, although both are quite rare. A bone scan or MRI can help diagnose these conditions. People with weakened immune systems may be at greater risk.

The constant throbbing or aching pain that occurs with a tumour or spinal infection may be quite severe throughout the day, worsen with rest, and be markedly different from the type of back pain that occasionally awakens you at night.

You have new symptoms or Excruciating Pain.

Always go to your doctor any time that you have pain so excruciating that you feel unbearable. You should also attend your doctor if you experience any new symptoms such as bowel or bladder problems, foot drop, or weakness as well as radiating pain, numbness or tingling or shooting pains in your legs.

You undergo a Serious Trauma:

If your back pain starts with a serious trauma like a bad fall or is exacerbated by some type of accident, you should attend your doctor. If your pain is unbearable and your doctor's is closed you will have to go to hospital.

Although most back pain does not require an imaging study such as an X ray or CT or MRI scan, in the case of trauma your doctor may need to use one of these tests to check for a possible vertebral fracture. Only your doctor can determine whether some type of vertebral fracture has occurred.

A vertebral fracture is generally not a serious problem and usually requires limited rest, time to heal, and appropriate treatment such as wearing a brace, appropriate activity restrictions and/or medicines. Once the fracture heals, your back should return to functioning normally and painlessly. A small percentage of spinal fractures are unstable and require surgery to repair.

You are Not Seeing Improvement.

If you have tried all the home remedies and various advice but have seen no improvement, attend your doctor first before getting help from another health care professional. A medical evaluation ensures that your back pain is not due to a serious or dangerous condition. After your medical evaluation rules out any significant problems, you can focus on getting better.

Conservative treatments for your back pain include home remedies or more formal medical treatment such as physiotherapy. A physiotherapy course usually is from six to eight weeks and you should attend your doctor for follow up when you finish.

Physiotherapy treatment can initially aggravate your back pain due to the increase in activity and physiological changes that treatment produces, but after a few weeks you should begin to feel some relief from your symptoms. If you do not notice improvements see your doctor.

Your Medications Are not Working

See your doctor in either of these medicine-related situations:

1. You experience any side effects to either prescription or over-the-counter medications: Your doctor may want to alter your dosage or switch you to another medication.

Herbs are becoming increasingly more popular but they are medicines too. Always tell your doctor whether you are combining herbal and prescription medicines. If you begin to experience side effects, your doctor may need to evaluate any drug interactions.

2. You are using drugs to self-medicate your back pain: Self-medicating in this sense includes such things as using more medication than is prescribed for you, using alcohol to treat your back pain, using someone else's medication, or using other substances or drugs to manage your pain.

Chapter 8: Back pain Prevention

Taking a few sensible precautions, such as leading a healthy lifestyle, can help prevent back pain and lower your risk of hurting your back. For example, you should:

- Take regular exercise
- Use a safe technique when lifting heavy objects
- Always maintain a good posture when sitting and standing

Lifting

One of the biggest causes of back injury at work is lifting or handling objects incorrectly.

Learning and following the correct method for lifting and handling heavy loads can help to prevent injury and avoid back pain.

Think before you lift

Plan the lift. Where is the load going to be placed? Use appropriate handling aids where possible. Will help be needed with the load? Remove obstructions, such as discarded wrapping materials. For long lifts, such as from floor to shoulder height, consider resting the load mid-way on a table or bench to change grip.

Keep the load close to the waist

Keep the load close to the waist for as long as possible while lifting. The distance of the load from the spine at waist height is an important factor in the overall load on the spine and back muscles. Keep the heaviest side of the load next to the body. If closely approaching the load is not possible, try to slide it towards the body before trying to lift it.

Adopt a stable position

Your feet should be apart with one leg slightly forward to maintain balance (alongside the load if it is on the ground). Be prepared to move your feet during the lift in order to maintain a stable posture. Wearing over-tight clothing or unsuitable footwear, such as heels or flip flops, may make this difficult.

Ensure a good hold on the load

Where possible; hug the load close to the body. This may be a better option than gripping it tightly with the hands only.

Do not bend your back

A slight bending of the back, hips and knees at the start of the lift is preferable to either fully flexing the back (stooping) or fully flexing the hips and knees, i.e. fully squatting.

Do not flex the back any further while lifting.

This can happen if the legs begin to straighten before starting to raise the load.

Do not twist

Avoid twisting the back or leaning sideways especially while the back is bent. Keep your shoulders level and facing the same direction as the hips. Turning by moving your feet is better than twisting and lifting at the same time.

Keep your head up

Keep your head up when handling the load. Look ahead, not down at the load once it has been held securely.

Move smoothly

Do not jerk or snatch the load as this can make it harder to keep control and can increase the risk of injury.

Know your limits

Do not lift or handle more than you can easily manage. There's a difference between what people can lift and what they can safely lift. If you are in doubt, seek advice or get help.

Lower down, and then adjust

Put the load down and then adjust. If you need to position the load precisely, put it down first, and then slide it into the desired position.

Sitting Posture

If you work in an office and use a computer, you can avoid injury by sitting in the right position and arranging your desk correctly.

Sitting in the wrong position can cause or aggravate back pain. Try to follow these simple tips to combat poor sitting habits:

- Sit up with your back straight and your shoulders down and back, elbows relaxed at your sides. Your buttocks should touch the back of your chair.
- Avoid crossing your legs. This weakens your core muscles and can lead to stiffness in your low back and pelvic area.
- Your feet should be firmly on the floor, but if it is more comfortable, use a footrest.
- Your thighs should be at right angles to your body or sloping slightly down.
- Rest your elbows and arms on your chair's armrests or desk, keeping your shoulders relaxed.
- When sitting in a chair that rolls and pivots, do not twist at the waist while sitting. Instead, turn your whole body.
- Do not sit in one position for long periods of time. Get up and move around at least every forty-five minutes, however, every twenty minutes is better. Do not forget to stretch.
- When standing up, move to the front of the seat of your chair. Stand up by straightening your legs. Avoid bending forward at your waist.

Support your back

Avoid back pain by adjusting your chair so that your lower back is properly supported. A correctly adjusted chair will reduce the strain on your back. Get one that is easily adjustable so that you can change the height, back position and tilt. Have your knees level with your hips. You may need a footrest for this.

Adjust your chair

Adjust your chair height so that you can use the keyboard with your wrists and forearms straight and level with the floor. This can help prevent repetitive strain injuries. Your elbows should be by the side of your body, so that the arm forms an L-shape at the elbow joint.

Place your screen at eye level

Your screen should be directly in front of you. A good guide is to place the monitor about an arm's length away, with the top of the screen roughly at eye level. To achieve this you may need to get a stand for your monitor. If the screen is too high or too low, you will have to bend your neck, which can be uncomfortable.

Make objects accessible

Position frequently used objects, such as your telephone or stapler, within easy reach. Avoid repeatedly stretching or twisting to reach things.

Avoid phone strain

If you spend a lot of time on the phone, try exchanging your handset for a headset. Repeatedly cradling the phone between your ear and shoulder can strain the muscles in your neck.

Keeping your back strong

Strengthening your back through exercise is one of the best ways to keep back pain at bay. It can also be very helpful in treating back pain.

Choose a low-impact, gentle exercise that will help strengthen the muscles in your back, without the risk of strain or sudden jolts. Swimming, yoga and Pilates are very good for improving flexibility and strength and once you feel your back is strong enough, you can graduate to something more energetic such as jogging, cycling or dancing.

Pick something you enjoy so that it is more likely to become a habit. You should aim to exercise three to five times a week for thirty minutes each time.

Stretching is another key way of strengthening your back. It can help to warm up the muscles in your back before starting to exercise and can even be helpful in preparing your back muscles prior to household chores or gardening. But the best way of maximising the benefits of stretching is to make them a part of your everyday routine.

Driving

Driving can prove a real challenge for backs, especially if you drive for extended periods of time.

- Sit with your buttocks touching the back of the seat. Adjust the seat so that your leg is slightly bent when you press a pedal to the floor.
- For maximum back support, adjust seat depth so the distance between the edge of the seat and the back of your knees is about two or three fingers wide.
- Your shoulders should be down and back against the backrest. They should remain in contact with the backrest when you turn the steering wheel.
- Adjust the angle of the backrest so that you can easily reach the steering wheel with your arms bent.
- If you feel your seat is not giving good support, try a rolled-up towel or lumbar roll in the small of your back.
- Adjust the tilt of the seat so that you can easily press the pedals down to the floor. Your thighs should rest lightly on the seat cushion without pressing on it.
- The top of the headrest should be aligned with the top of your head. Adjust the angle to allow under an inch of space between your head and the headrest.
- While driving, keep your chin in and do not grip the wheel too hard. Relax your shoulders and keep your head upright.
- To reduce the risk of lower back pain, avoid sitting still for lengthy periods and stop regularly to walk and stretch.
- Try to avoid twisting when getting out of the car. Turn your whole body towards the door; lower your feet to the ground and then stand up.

Computers

Computers are probably the biggest problem when it comes to back or neck strain. Ensuring your workspace is set up correctly will help in reducing the potential for harm:

- Your keyboard should be directly in front of you. A keyboard that is off-centre can cause bad posture.
- Turn your chair sideways to check that your elbow is level with the spacebar for the correct height.
- If your keyboard is at the proper height, you should be able to keep your wrists straight while typing. This posture will reduce the risk of injury.
- A palm or wrist support can help during rest periods from using the keyboard. Place the support under your palms, not your wrists.
- Your mouse should be close to your keyboard. You should be able to keep your wrist straight, shoulders relaxed and elbows by your side while using it.
- If you need to look back and forth between your monitor and documents, place your hard copy in such a way so as to avoid twisting your neck.
- Consider a document holder, which should be placed close to and at the same height as the screen.
- Place your phone close to you to avoid repetitive reaching.
- Avoid cradling the phone between your ear and shoulder as this can cause neck pain and stiffness. Consider a headset or speaker phone.

Laptop use tips

- Use a separate keyboard and mouse so that the laptop can be put on a stand and the screen opened at eye level.
- Use your laptop on a stable base where there is support for your arms, and not on your lap.
- Take regular breaks. If you are moving, there's a lot less stress on your muscles and joints.
- Adopt good sitting posture with lower back support, and ensure that other desk equipment is within reach.
- Get into good habits before the aching starts. Neck, shoulder and back problems gradually build up over time.

Bad posture is inevitable because of the way laptops are designed. The main problem is the keyboard being attached to the screen.

You need the screen at arm's length but you need the keyboard near you, so you push the laptop further back, then your hands stretch out, then you hunch your shoulders. That creates bad posture.

The average human head weighs quite a lot. If it is in the ideal position, balanced above the shoulders, it is fine but when you use a laptop, your ears are further forward than your shoulders. That is like taking a weight and holding it out at arm's length.

The load through your spine is much greater and, even worse; it is a static load as you are not moving. This causes neck, upper back and arm problems.

Fitness

If you are not fit you are much more likely to damage your back as it will not be as flexible as it should be. Therefore, fitness is important in the prevention of back pain.

Weight Control

Being overweight puts too much strain on all weight bearing joints, including those of the spine. This will increase the curve of the spine (Lordosis) and will also increase the rate of wear and tear on those joints.

Being overweight means that you are not fit and not being fit means that you are more likely to suffer from backache.

Mobility

Good posture is not possible unless you have a mobile spine and good muscle tone. The flexibility of the spine and the strength of its supporting muscles are essential functions, without which the spine loses some of its shock absorbing capacity and is more vulnerable to injury.

Joints must be moved to keep them mobile and the muscles, both abdominal (tummy) and back, must be used to keep them strong. For many of us our lifestyle is not conducive to maintaining good mobile joints and good strong muscles and so exercise is necessary to keep the joints and muscles in good working order.

General exercise including swimming, walking and many sports help to do this as well as helping our overall fitness level.

Exercises that stretch and strengthen the muscles of your abdomen and spine can help prevent back problems. If your back and abdominal muscles are strong, it will help you to maintain good posture and keep your spine in its correct position.

Warm up your muscles with light aerobic activity like brisk walking before doing any strengthening or stretching. Wear close clothing to make it easier to do the exercises. Stop doing any exercise that causes pain until you have spoken with your health care provider.

Posture

Posture can be divided into two categories: Static posture is the position of your body when you are stationary. Examples of static posture are standing and sitting. Dynamic posture is the position of your body as it moves.

Understanding what healthy static and dynamic postures look and feel like may help you prevent back pain episodes from occurring as well as managing your back pain when it does occur.

Static Postures

Even though you are not moving, static postures can place unnecessary pressures on your spine if you assume an unhealthy position. People spend a great deal of time standing, sitting, and lying down during a typical day. Understanding how to be in these positions comfortably may play an important role in your total back health.

As an individual, you have a unique standing position that is efficient, comfortable, and healthy for your back. The ideal standing posture supports your body in a balanced, upright alignment with minimal use of muscle energy and no perception of strain. A good way to assess your current standing posture is to stand sidewise in front of a full-length mirror.

If you have another mirror available, you can place the two mirrors at an angle so that you can look straight ahead into one while getting a side view of yourself from the other. Using two mirrors helps you avoid having to turn your neck to the side to observe your posture. As you look in the mirror, allow yourself to assume a posture that is an exaggeration of your normal standing posture. For instance, if you tend to slump your shoulders, slump them more. Or, if your stomach tends to stick out, push it out more. Although your exaggerated posture is not your everyday posture, it can help you identify problems as you go through the following list. As you assume your exaggerated posture, ask yourself these questions:

- **Are my knees locked or bent?**
Your knees should be relatively straight, but not entirely locked.

- **What's going on with my lower back, pelvis, and abdomen?**

Ideally, your waistline (representing your pelvis) is fairly level: Your lower back exhibits only a mild curve and your abdomen is "tucked in."

- **Are my shoulders slumped over?**

Ideally, your shoulders are not rounded forward and slumped over. Generally, your shoulders should be in a straight line with your torso.

- **Are my head and neck tilted forward from my shoulders?**

Your head should be fairly centred over the top of your chest and in a level position. Your neck should appear fairly straight, with a slight forward curve. As you check yourself out in the mirror, you may notice some unhealthy aspects of your standing position. See whether your stance has any of these features:

The military stance:

This is the stance that you probably assumed as a child when you were told to "Stand up straight." In this position, you stand as straight, tall, and rigid as you can. Even though the military stance may look good, it is not healthy for your back. It can actually cause your lower back to curve more (causing your stomach to stick out) and your head to tip backwards over your neck, which strains the ligaments and muscles of your upper back.

Slumped posture:
In the slumped posture, your head is tilted forward, your shoulders are slumped forward and down, and your stomach sticks out, increasing the curve of your lower back. Slumped posture may irritate and put excessive strain on structures in your lower back. The tilted head and curve of your spine can also cause neck pain.

Adopting healthy standing habits

A healthy standing position may feel uncomfortable at first, especially if you have been "practicing" an unhealthy standing posture for 30 or 40 years (or more).

To practice a healthy standing position, stand against a wall with your heels approximately two inches away from it. (Standing slightly away from the wall allows room for your buttocks.) Do a pelvic tilt — move the small of your back toward the wall by tilting your pelvis. Keep your knees slightly bent and making sure not to lock them in a straight position.

If you must stand for an extended length of time, be sure to use a footrest. Simply placing one foot up on a short stool or stack of books gives you a healthier standing posture. Be sure to alternate your feet every once in a while. This position reduces the curve in your lower back and decreases the strain on the facet joints in your lower spine.

Wearing high heels increases the curve of your lower back, possibly placing more strain on it.

You can decrease strain on your back simply by placing commonly used household items at eye level. Doing so helps you avoid bending and leaning throughout the day as you use these items. If you are standing for a long period of time, try to move about and alternate your position frequently. You can change positions to keep your muscles and spine relaxed.

Sitting

Sitting, especially in the same position for an extended time, is thought to be more stressful on your back than standing, lying down, and, in some cases, lifting. Sitting is stressful on your back because your muscles have to work harder to keep you upright and stable. If your back is not well supported while sitting, your muscles fatigue quickly. When this happens, you tend to slouch in order to give your muscles a break. Slouching causes your centre of gravity to shift forward and your pelvis to rotate backward, which places your lower spine in an unnatural position.

This unnatural position means that the discs of your lumbar spine must bear the weight of your entire upper body unevenly. Studies have shown that pressure between discs increases with sitting. Although certain well-designed chairs can help decrease distress on your spine, people often sit on the edge of their chairs out of habit, which defeats the design of the chair.

Slumped posture: If you are sitting posture is slumped, then your lower back tends to be rounded out, your chest is depressed inward, your upper back is rounded forward, and your neck is arched backward in order to keep your head level. Your head probably feels like it is projecting out in front of your chest rather than being balanced above your torso.

Slumped sitting greatly increases the pressure on your lower back. In this position, the middle and upper joints of your neck tend to be crammed together because of the increased backward arching. The muscles of your neck and shoulders are also overworked in this position. After sitting in this position for an extended period of time, you may also notice difficulties straightening up into a standing position.

Tense sitting: In this type of sitting, you sustain a certain level of tension in your muscles due to your back being unsupported, being in a stressful situation, or simply by habit. People who engage in tense sitting are often not even aware that their bodies are tense. Tense sitting can occur either in conjunction with unhealthy posture or even with healthy posture for sitting. For example, you may maintain a healthy posture while having virtually all the muscles in your body in a state of low-level tension. Becoming aware of muscle tension and practicing relaxation, can help reduce this muscle tension.

Sitting too long: If you are like most people, your most common posture in the course of a day is sitting. The problem is that your body is not designed to be in this position for an extended period of time without any movement. Even when you are sitting correctly, it is important for your body to move about regularly. Sitting for long periods of time puts strain on the structures of your back, including the muscles.

Crossing your legs: Another common posture is to cross your

legs while sitting. For short periods of time, this posture is comfortable and allows your muscles to relax. Staying in this position for an extended period of time, however, causes some of the same problems as sitting too long. Also, crossing your legs while sitting in a chair that does not provide support causes you to hold a slumped or tense sitting posture.

The first rule of healthy sitting is to become aware of whether you experience any of the unhealthy patterns described in the preceding section. The following healthy sitting guidelines can help you sit more comfortably and reduce the stress on your lower back:

- Position your pelvis: Healthy sitting involves paying attention to the position of your pelvis — it affects the position of your lower back and your entire upper body. To position your pelvis properly, move your tail bone back as far as possible in the chair with your upper body tilting forward (imagine tucking your buttocks into the back of the chair).

- After you tuck your pelvis into the back of the chair, bring your body into the upright position. This move repositions your pelvis into a healthy posture. You may need to adjust this position slightly (for example, rolling your pelvis slightly forward or backward)

- As you become familiar with a healthy sitting position, you can change your position frequently and keep stressful forces on your lower back to a minimum. The primary goal is to keep your pelvis, chest, and head aligned whether you are sitting back, up, or forward. Thus, as your upper torso leans backwards, your lower body should tilt upward to maintain the proper posture or angle between your upper and lower body.

- If you are sitting with your pelvis back in the chair (and your upper body slightly backward), you may want to place a small footstool (these are often designed with a slant to fit your feet) or telephone book under your feet. Using a footstool helps raise your knees slightly above hip level, which puts your pelvis in a healthy position.

- If you are sitting on the edge of a chair, you should keep your knees lower than your hips, move your legs wider apart than normally, and position one foot forward and the other foot farther back on the floor. Use a good chair for sitting: Getting a chair designed for healthy sitting is very important, especially if the chair is one you sit in for extended periods of time on a regular basis, such as in the office. The more you sit, the more your body takes on the shape of the particular chair you use.

- Use proper supports in unsupported chairs: If you must use a chair that does not provide proper support, you can take steps to improve your sitting position. First, if the chair does not provide support for your lower back, you can put a rolled-up towel or small pillow across the small of your back to help keep the natural curve of your lower back while sitting. Many lumbar support pillows are available commercially.

- Second, if you tend to sink down in the chair (as often happens in worn-out restaurant booths or soft couches), you can put a folded towel or even a book under your buttocks to fill in part of the seat you are sinking into. Take breaks and move around: One of the best ways to keep your back healthy while sitting is to take frequent breaks and move around. Taking breaks is sometimes quite a challenge, though, especially when you become engrossed in a task and do not realize that you have been sitting in the same position for two or three hours. If you are prone to sitting too long, try setting a timer for about every 30 minutes to remind you to get up and take a break. When you do, try such activities as walking around

- Choosing the best chair for you depends upon such factors as your body shape and the type of work you will be doing while sitting in the chair. The following are some general guidelines related to obtaining a proper chair:

    o A good chair supports and maintains your spine in its natural shape as you sit in it. Particularly, the curve in the small of your back should not be either excessive or reduced, but rather maintained in its natural form. If you are not using a chair at a desk, try one that tilts back slightly with a footrest to support your feet. The height of a desk chair should be easy to adjust. If the seat of your chair is too high, the curve of your lower back increases to an unhealthy position, your feet almost dangle, and the muscles of your upper and lower back strain.

109

- o Most good chairs have a hydraulic mechanism for changing height. Most high-quality office chairs provide specific lumbar support for your lower back — something you want to be sure you get.

- When the muscles of your lower back are not properly supported, they contract. This low-level muscle contraction, when sustained for many hours, causes muscle fatigue and spasm, which may lead to pain. Avoid a chair that you "sink into. "A soft chair actually causes the muscles in your lower back to be tenser as they attempt to provide your spine with the support that the chair lacks. The chair should have a curved front edge. A sharp edge that puts undue pressure on your upper legs can decrease blood flow to your thighs and lower legs.

- The chair should transfer the majority of your weight to your buttocks rather than your thighs while you are sitting. Some chairs are so straight-backed that they "push" your upper body forward, causing pressure on your thighs. If possible, choose a chair with armrests. Armrests can help decrease the tension and fatigue on your neck and shoulders. Armrests can also help you stabilize the chair when making the transition from sitting to standing and vice versa.

Lying Down

Although a great deal of advice is available on proper sleeping positions, the research is not all that clear on whether different sleeping positions impact your back pain. It appears that sleeping positions may be an individual thing: For you, it may be important, and for others, it does not matter.

Lying on your stomach:

Lying on your stomach increases the curve of your lower back. If sleeping on your stomach is a difficult position for you to give up, you can try to straighten out your spine by placing a pillow or towel under your pelvis.

Lying Flat on your Back:

Lying flat on your back with your legs outstretched increases the curve in your lower back and may cause stress to that area. If you prefer to sleep on your back, you can support your hips by bending your knees and placing a pillow underneath them. Doing so places your lower back in a natural, comfortable position.

Foetal Position:

Using the foetal position: Like many other people with back pain, you may find that the foetal position is the most comfortable. In this position, you lie on your side with both hips and knees bent equally.

Placing a small pillow between your knees may make you even more comfortable. Also, you can put a small pillow under your head and neck to fill the space between your head and shoulders.

Being aware of the couch:

Your couch can be thought of as a small-size soft bed. Therefore, lying down on the couch (to sleep, watch TV, or read) may cause the same stresses as lying on a soft bed. Instead, you may want to lie on your back on the floor with your knees bent over some pillows or a chair. You can place a small pillow under your neck to support your head.

Choosing a mattress:

A well-made mattress and box spring set should last between seven and fifteen years, depending upon the quality and how you take care of the bed. Part of proper bed maintenance includes turning the mattress end to end and upside down every month for the first few months so that it adjusts evenly to your body weight. After that time, you should turn the mattress every couple of months. Of course, if you have a back pain problem, get help to turn your mattress and use proper lifting techniques.

Because you spend about one-third of your life in bed, you should invest wisely. Unfortunately, it is not possible to "try out" a bed for a few weeks to decide whether you like it. Even so, you should spend five or ten minutes seeing how it feels in the showroom. Most mattresses use a spring coil construction. Mattresses can vary greatly in terms of the number and thickness of the coil springs. Other mattresses use things like "baffles" and other design features in conjunction with the coil springs. Finding a bed that is comfortable for you is a highly individual choice. You want a mattress and box spring set that is neither too firm nor too soft but provides enough support to keep your back in its natural curves.

Dynamic Posture

Dynamic postures involve the position that your body takes while it is in motion. Movement requires that your muscles, ligaments, and bones all work together in a coordinated fashion. Proper dynamic posture is moving in such a way that places the least amount of stress on your body to complete the required motion, and using the posture most likely to prevent injury to your spine.

Paying attention to proper dynamic posture is a little more difficult than static posture because you may not have as much time to plan ahead. As with standing and sitting, you need to evaluate your walking posture for unhealthy habits.

A good way to assess your walking is to watch yourself walk from the side in a mirror. As with assessing your sitting and standing postures, exaggerate your movements. If you tend to walk with your head forward or your stomach out, do it more. If you walk fairly loose and casually, loosen up even more. And, if you walk in a fast and more rigid manner, exaggerate those qualities.

Understanding what type of unhealthy patterns of walking you are likely to engage in helps you correct them and adapt the healthy walking patterns we describe later in this chapter. The following walking patterns may put more stress and strain on your lower back:

Stomach-out walking:
Increasing the forward arch of your lower back, along with stretching out your lower stomach, causes your pelvis to tilt forward as you walk. This alignment can aggravate low-back pain. In this unhealthy walking posture, you tend to walk with your abdomen leading far out in front of the rest of your body.

Head-forward walking:
Head-forward walking is generally caused by looking down at the ground directly in front of you while you walk. When you do so, you also put your chest in a depressed position, which puts stress on your neck, shoulders, and lower back due to unhealthy alignment. It also results in poor breathing and overall endurance.

Loose walking:
Loose walking is characterized by a tendency to be wobbly and engage in extraneous movements of the joints of your legs, arms, neck, and back. You may be prone to this type of walking if you have a tendency toward joint instability and muscle weakness.

Stiff walking:
The opposite of loose walking, stiff walking can be due to such things as being tense and uptight, having a fear of falling or re-injury, or a concern about making your back pain worse. People

who stiff-walk look like they have a corset or brace from their neck to their lower back (or, in more severe cases, from their head to their toes). This type of walking looks very robotic.

Stiff walking causes your muscles to work too hard as they try to prevent any motion from occurring around your neck and back. This muscle over activity tends to pull all the joints of your body together in a state of total body contraction. Stiff walking causes you to tire rapidly due to the amount of energy you expend to maintain rigidity. Stiff walking actually increases the probability of injury and pain flare-ups in your back.

Heel-pounding walking:
This type of walking pattern is characterized by a heavy heel- or foot-strike each time you take a step. It is as if you are pounding out a beat as you walk. This type of walking sends shock waves from your foot to your leg and up to your pelvic and spinal joints. The shock waves create extra stress throughout these body parts. This type of walking is usually developed through habit and is more exaggerated when you are in a hurry, emotionally upset, barefoot, or wearing heels that are either hard or spiked.

Stress walking:
Stress walking is characterized by taking fast, choppy steps with your upper body held forward and your head down. Similar to the heel-pounding walk, stress walking transmits shock waves from your lower body to your pelvis and spine. Stress walking also includes total body muscle tension, especially around areas of pain such as your lower back. You may stress-walk as a matter of habit, and it gets worse when you are under emotional

pressure.

Becoming a healthy walker

Before attempting to adopt healthy walking, identify whether you are exhibiting any of the unhealthy patterns we describe in the preceding list. Doing so helps you focus your practice of the healthy walking techniques. The following are some tips for healthy walking:

Make your pelvis level:

Keep your hips and lower back in a stable position as you walk. This tip involves doing a slight pelvic tilt as you walk. Imagine a straight line coming directly out of the centre of your stomach or bellybutton as you walk. Generally, that line points at a downward angle. In order to get a slight pelvic tilt, imagine shifting the line up slightly. Doing this slight shift while you walk results in a tilt that brings your pelvis to a more level position and makes walking easier on your spine.

Release tension as you walk:

Use breathing techniques while you walk to keep the muscles of your body, including your back, in a fairly relaxed state. Each time you slowly exhale while you walk, think about releasing any tightness that is holding your body rigid. This technique can help prevent stiff walking, stress walking, and heel pounding.

Keep your head light:

This one may sound funny, but thinking in terms of keeping your head and neck light on your shoulders as you walk can help you walk better. You should allow your head and neck to relax and simply balance on top of your shoulders. This helps decrease any tension you may be carrying in your shoulders or neck.

Use a soft landing:
As you walk, think about your legs moving smoothly and your feet landing softly as they touch the ground with each step. The most important thing is to reduce the amount of pounding and the shock waves generated throughout your lower body. Simply focus on landing each foot more quietly, softly, and smoothly. As you practice smooth walking, you can do it efficiently while walking as fast as you desire.

The type of shoes you wear can also help you walk more smoothly and decrease heel pounding. Especially good shoes are running shoes with a snug heel, room for the front of your foot, proper support, and excellent cushioning.

Walk smoothly:
As you walk, allow your head and trunk to be relatively upright in order to maintain a healthy posture and improve breathing. Limit any extra movement of your hips, and keep your head from tipping forward, backward, or off to either side. There should not be much twisting between your various body parts, such as your upper and lower body. Visualize your face, shoulders, chest, and hips being in a relatively stable position and facing forward while you walk. Healthy walking involves a smooth motion of the muscles of your legs and feet.

Buying a pair of shoes
The type of shoes that you wear might impact how your back feels while standing and walking. Your shoes determine how

your lower body interacts with the ground in two ways: positioning and transmission of shock waves. No matter what type of shoe you wear, from athletic to dressy, pay attention to some basics of healthy footwear:

The part of the shoe that surrounds your heel (the heel counter) should be stable enough to hold your heel upright while you stand and walk. The heel counter should be made of reinforced and durable material. If the heel counter is weak, it allows your heel to move either inward or outward, increasing strain on your legs and your lower back.

The heel of the shoe is the platform under the bones of your heel. The heel should be well padded to absorb shock and be elevated slightly above the ball of your foot. The width of the heel should be equal to the width of the heel counter in order to help distribute the shock from walking. Hard and dense heels increase the amount of shock transmitted from your legs to your back. Spiked heels can cause an unstable effect on the legs that may increase muscle tension in the lower back. Beware of heels that have worn unevenly, because they can cause you to walk and stand unevenly and increase the stress on your spine.

A shoe should have a reasonable amount of flexibility at the ball of the foot to provide a smooth motion while walking. If the sole of the shoe is too rigid, it does not "give" when you try to bend it. A stiff sole is not only uncomfortable but causes you to walk in an unnatural and unhealthy way. On the other hand, a sole that is too flexible and soft does not give your feet the proper support that they need (especially in the arches).

The insole is the inside, flat part of the shoe and extends from the toes to the heel. The insole of your shoe should provide comfortable support to the heel and arch of your foot. As you look inside one of your shoes, you should see a contour that matches the shape of the bottom of your foot. A good insole has a build-up of material to support the arch. If this build-up is not there, your feet tend to fall inward and flatten out, putting your lower body into a state of misalignment that increases pressure on your lower spine.

The toe box is that part of the shoe that surrounds your toes. The toe box should allow enough room for your toes to move around while providing adequate support on either side of your foot. The side support should prevent your toes from moving excessively from side to side. The toe box should not in any way cramp or crunch your toes. You should not feel the top of your toes hitting the roof of the toe box.

Chapter 9: BACK to Work

If your back pain has kept you from your job, returning to work can be daunting. You may doubt your ability to do your job, especially if your work is physical, and you may wonder whether you can spend eight hours at work — not to mention your commute — without resting your back. On the other hand, returning to work can be very rewarding. Work gives you a sense of purpose and gives your life routine. Shedding the discomfort and unpredictability of pain is a relief in itself.

Work gives you a sense of self-esteem and identity (not to mention your wages).

A back pain injury that disables you from work is not just a physical blow to your body, but also a mental and emotional one. The longer you are disabled from work because of back pain, the more your pain affects you emotionally and within your social circles.

Studies indicate that if you have been absent from work because of back pain disability for six months, the chances of your going back to work are about seventy-five percent. After twelve months, those chances decline to fifty percent. If you have been disabled from work due to back pain for more than two years, your chances of ever returning to work approach zero. Keep in mind that these statistics are based on large groups of injured workers and may not predict what can happen to you as an individual. But knowing these statistics can help ensure that you do not become a "statistic." *(G.B.J Anderson, "The Epidemiology of Spinal Disorders," in The Adult Spine edited by J.W. Frymoyer, (New York: Raven Press, 1991).*

Jobs that require lifting and bending:

If your job requires heavy lifting, pulling, or carrying, the repetitive motion and strain can lead to lumbar disc disease. Many studies show a significant association between lifting, pushing, pulling, and low-back pain and sciatica. Particularly important is the posture that you adopt during lifting moves. One of the worst positions is lifting while twisting at the same time.

Laboratory experiments show that this type of movement can produce tears in the structures that surround the disc. If you lift and twist improperly at work, you can expect to have a two- to threefold increase in the risk of lumbar disc herniation. If your job involves heavy labour, a number of factors can determine if you have a back injury: the amount of weight you are lifting, the frequency of lifting, and your lifting technique. Your overall physical fitness is also significant. If you exceed your overall physical capacity for lifting on a regular basis, your risk of low-back injury increases as much as four times. Although your maximum lifting load is highly variable depending upon your physical condition, generally, the maximum lifting load is thirty to thirty-five pounds for women and fifty to sixty pounds for men.

If you regularly lift objects that are much heavier than these guidelines, you are at risk. Consider getting help or using some other technique to avoid lifting, such as using a cart or dolly. Using proper posture techniques and staying in good physical condition can help prevent back injury. If you are already disabled from heavy lifting because of a back injury, you need to decide if you will ever be able to return to that type of work.

Exposure to vibration

Prolonged exposure to vibration, especially that caused by motor vehicles, creates a significantly higher risk for low-back pain problems, sciatica, and disc herniation. Laboratory studies have shown that the frequency of vibration that is stressful to your back is similar to the vibration you experience when driving in a car. If you are exposed to vibration during work, then your risk for developing one of these conditions is two to three times that of the general population, according to studies.

Also, you are at greater risk for a back injury if you commute to work more than twenty miles per day or drive a truck as part of your workday. In fact, if you spend more than half your job driving a motor vehicle, you are three times more likely than the average worker to suffer a herniated disc. A sitting position places additional stress on your back.

As your spine is exposed to vibration in the sitting position, your spine is exposed to greater stress. Vibration also fatigues the muscles that support your spine. You can take steps to reduce vibration to your spine by driving a car with a softer suspension, trying not to drive over rough terrain and using a seat cushion and/or back brace that provides proper support. If you are on disability from a job that exposes you to vibration, you need to take special steps to safely return to that type of work.

Sitting

If your job requires a great deal of sitting, you have an increased risk for a back injury. Sedentary occupations in general are not good for your back because sitting puts great pressure on the disc between your vertebrae.

Commuting

Commuting by car, bus or train causes you to be in a sitting position while your spine is subjected to vibration. The following tips can help you as you commute. Watch your position: Be sure that your sitting position is upright with your pelvis tucked back. Move your seat up so that you can easily reach the pedals and do not have to stretch your lower extremities. Reclining the backrest about 5–15 degrees can also be helpful.

Do some easy commuter stretches: As you drive, occasionally push your arms straight on the steering wheel to help decompress your lower back and pelvis. You can also periodically arch your lower back forward and away from the back of the seat while doing a slight stretch. Check your seat: If you are driving in your own car or flying in a plane, check your seat to see whether you need better back support. This can be obtained by such things as using a lumbar roll, repositioning yourself, and repositioning the seat. You can also take weight off your spine by using an arm rest.

Avoid keeping your head turned to one side: While you are driving, avoid keeping your head turned to one side for too long.

This can cause muscle tension beginning in your neck and also occurring in your lower back. If you do notice tension from turning your head, look in the opposite direction for a few seconds to help balance yourself out. Stay relaxed: Being in stop-and-go traffic can be one of the worst situations for tensing up. To combat stress, try playing relaxing music or take a few deep breaths, exhaling slowly each time. Take breaks on a long drive: If you are driving for a long time, take breaks and get out of the car.

Choosing to return to work

Even though you may be motivated to return to work after a low-back injury, several challenges may get in your way. Here are some of the likely factors that may cause difficulty:

Legal intervention:

If legal aspects are involved in your work injury case, this can act as a blockade for return to work. Legal action often creates an adversarial relationship between you and your employer. You may consciously or unconsciously believe that returning to work will hurt your legal case, which ultimately affects your ability to successfully return to work.

Job dissatisfaction:

Recent research indicates that how much you like your job (or do not like it) may be one of the most important risk factors for getting a back injury that results in disability. This makes sense: The more you like your job and the more satisfying it is, the more motivated you will be to return to it regardless of back pain.

Disability income:

The type and amount of your disability income can also affect your return to work. For instance, if your disability income closely approximates your normal take-home pay, you are likely to be on disability longer after a back injury. This makes sense: If you are not receiving enough income to support yourself while on disability because of a back injury, you are more likely to return to any type of work in order to support your family.

Psychological factors:

Psychological factors such as occupational stress, job dissatisfaction, anxiety, and depression are all risk factors for back injury and pain. Also, any of these psychological factors can delay or even prevent your return to work after a back injury.

Inappropriate medical care:

Receiving inappropriate medical care for your back problem can delay your return to work.

Inappropriate medical care can include such elements as too much bed rest, inactivity, or overmedication.

Chronic health problems:

If you have other health problems aside from your back injury, you are less likely to be able to return to work. Your back injury may be "the straw that breaks the camel's back," in terms of your physical ability to perform your job duties.

Poor labour market:

If the labour market in your area is particularly bad, this can delay your return to work due to a decrease in the number of options. This is especially the case if you will not be returning to your previous job or career.

Limited education/job skills:

If your education is limited and your jobs have always been in heavy physical labour, you may have difficulty returning to work after a significant back injury.

In the past, your general physician — with very little influence from outside agencies — decided whether you returned to work. This is not the case today. Returning to work most likely requires the coordinated involvement of healthcare providers, governmental officials and programs, providers of rehabilitation services, medical utilization review organizations, solicitors, your employer among others. Getting all of these systems and people working together toward successfully returning you to work can be quite a daunting task.

The decision to try and begin the process to return to work

ultimately will be yours. You have many options in your decision to return to work:

Return to work with no restrictions:

Under this option you decide to return to your previous job without any restrictions relative to your back injury. You return on a full-time, full-duty capacity.

Return to work with restricted duties:

Under this option, you decide to return to your previous job, but with appropriate medical restrictions for your back injury. You can be restricted from bending, lifting, and twisting. You may also be subject to a weight lifting restriction. In addition, you may begin working on a part-time basis. When you return to work after a period of prolonged disability, it is always a good idea to return part-time with appropriate medical restrictions.

Unfortunately, some employers do not allow this type of return to work. If it is possible in your case, try to return to work on a part-time basis initially. Easing back into your job allows your body to become accustomed to the increased physical demands of returning to work and to gradually increase your work endurance. For example, a part-time schedule may be three hours per day, five days per week or four to five hours per day, three days per week.

Pursuing vocational rehabilitation:

Under this option, you and your doctor decide that your back injury precludes you from returning to your previous job. For instance, if you were an auto-mechanic and performed repetitive bending and lifting throughout your day, a serious back injury may preclude you from ever going back to that occupation. You may choose to pursue vocational rehabilitation to learn a new job within your medical restrictions such as a more sedentary job without bending or lifting.

Return to work is not indicated:

Under this option, you and your doctors decide that returning to work is not an option given your back injury. Given your age, the type of back injury and resulting medical restrictions, it may not be realistic or even appropriate for you to try and return to any type of work. Therefore, permanent disability and retirement would be recommended.

Returning to work.

A return to work program includes anything you and your doctor can do to increase the chances that you can successfully return to work and stay there. Some of these things are done prior to returning to work, while others are done in the early phases of your return to work.

Physical Reconditioning:

Part of preparing to return to work should include physically reconditioning your body to be able to complete your job tasks. Deconditioning can result in a loss of muscle strength and endurance, decrease aerobic capacity and mobility, or inability to coordinate your movements properly.

Physical reconditioning prepares your body to do your work activities. If you return to work prior to your body being physically ready, you increase the chances of experiencing another back injury and more disability. The better shape you are in, the more likely you can successfully return to work.

Understand your body and your back:

Body mechanics involve how you position and move your body, especially related to your back. Using proper and safe body mechanics helps decrease any stress on your lower back and prevent re-injury.

Pacing:

When you pace yourself, you take regular breaks throughout your workday in order to prevent a build-up of stress on your spine. If your job requires extended sitting, you should take regular breaks to stand up, walk around and do some stretching exercises. If your job requires bending and lifting, then you take regular breaks from that activity.

Setting Limits:

When you return to work, be sure to set appropriate limits based on your physical capabilities to protect your spine. You may limit the amount of bending, lifting and twisting you are doing. You may also limit the amount of repetitive spinal movements done at one time. Sometimes setting limits can be difficult when your supervisor is requesting you to complete a certain task 'as quickly as possible'. It is at these times that you must be assertive and protect your back and prevent re-injury. Trying to save a few minutes by doing a task quickly is not worth risking another episode of disability.

Prepare for flare-ups:

You can usually expect flare-ups in your back pain after you do return to work due to the increased physical demands on your body. If you plan on flare-ups, you won't be surprised or overly concerned if they do occur. If your flare-up seems to go beyond something temporary, discuss it with your doctor. A common pattern in patients that return to work is 'three steps forward one step back'. Your work abilities and back pain will improve followed by a slight regression. Do not be concerned if you notice this pattern; it is fairly common.

Returning to the Office:

<u>Avoid keeping your head down:</u>

When sitting at your desk, or when standing over the copy machine, avoid the head-down position for an extended period of time. Pointing your head down places your neck and back in an unhealthy position.

Reposition yourself frequently: Push your pelvis back in your chair, avoid crossing your legs and use a chair that supports your spine.

Stretching at your desk:

Sit up in a tall relaxed, upright manner with your hands on your thighs to take the weight off your spine. Breathe in through your nose as you take this position, stretching yourself tall. As you exhale through your mouth, allow your head to gradually release forward. As you allow your head to release forward, you can think of the bones of your spine as the links of a chain. Allow each link to release sequentially, one at a time, from top to bottom. Stop lowering your body either when you feel ready to inhale or you achieve an adequate stretching sensation in your back. At this point release your body a little further as you inhale and then exhale again.

Continue this breathing pattern, releasing your body a little further each time you exhale. You should feel a release of tension in your neck, middle back and lower back. Temporary changes in your blood pressure may occur when doing this exercise that may cause dizziness, do not stand up immediately afterwards.

Spine release rotation:

After doing the forward stretch, bring one arm to the outside of the opposite knee and turn so that you can reach your other arm over the back of your chair. Gently turn your head, shoulders, and spine as far as you comfortably can in this same direction. Do this while keeping your knees straight ahead.

You should feel a comfortable and gentle stretch of your back. Do not worry if you notice little 'clicking' sound coming from your spine, these are normal. Each time you exhale, you can allow your arms to twist your back a little further, as you feel comfortable. After you inhale and exhale between one and three times, unwind slowly to the front position. Repeat the process in the opposite direction.

This is a gentle stretch and should not be done to the point of causing pain or discomfort.

Chapter 10: Back to Sport

Sporting activities can often be the first things to go after you suffer from a back pain problem. You may feel afraid of re-injury or that your spine can't take the pressure of sport involvement. For some of us, sport plays a huge part in our lives and the absence of it can often lead to depression, sleep disruption, muscle weakness and more back pain.

You can do many things to increase the safety of getting involved in sports and decrease the risk of injury to your back. Obviously some sporting activities carry more risk than others but certainly the benefits of participation in most cases outweigh the associated risks.

Prevention:

Warming up: Whether or not you have a problem with back pain, your body needs to warm up before engaging in any sporting activity. When you warm up, your heart rate increases, as does your circulation. This allows your muscles to react quickly without straining.

You can complete a warm up in a variety of ways: walking, cycling on a stationary bike or a few minutes on a treadmill. This should take no more than five to ten minutes. At the end of your warm-up, your heart rate should be elevated and you should be perspiring very slightly.

Warming up is crucial to being able to stretch your muscles to their limits without strain. If you try to stretch prior to warming up, you risk injuring your muscles just from the stretching activity. Concentrate your stretching program on the parts of your body that will be under the most stress while you are playing. For example before playing tennis, focus on stretching the muscles of your arms, legs, shoulders and lower back.

You may be tempted to bounce as you stretch in order to increase your range of motion but bouncing may injure your muscles. Simply stretch a particular muscle group to the end of its range and hold the position. You should sense a muscle 'pulling' while stretching, but never pain or tearing.

Do your stretching exercises slowly and gradually, always exhaling as you stretch. Hold each stretch for twenty seconds minimum to sixty seconds maximum.

Cooling Down: The cool down is probably the most neglected area of safe sporting. The rationale behind cooling down after the sport is to return your body gradually to its usual resting state. Cooling down allows your heart rate, circulatory system, muscle tension and respiration to return to normal slowly and gradually. Cool down activities include light walking, slow biking or gentle swimming.

When you engage in strenuous activity, your muscles contract and lactic acid may build up in your muscles and cause muscle pain if not given a chance to dissipate. When you do your cool-down stretch, contracted muscles return to normal, and lactic acid is carried away. The cool-down stretch also helps prevent muscle pain later on.

Risks:

Understanding the potential dangers of a particular sport is essential. Four types of movements/postures can exacerbate your back pain problem. These movements and postures are:

Flexion: Flexion is simply bending forward from a standing position. Flexion puts additional stress on the discs of your lumbar spine. The effects of repeated flexion can be cumulative, the stress of bending forty or fifty times during a game can add up to an irritation of your disc problem.

Extension: Extension is the opposite of flexion. Extension is a medical term for arching or bending backwards. Extension movements put stress on the facet joints of your lower back because when you arch backwards, the facet joints of your lower back are brought closer together. As with flexion, the results of repeated extension can be cumulative. For example in tennis , you hyper-extend your back when you serve, you may not notice the effects of a single serve but thirty to forty serves can result in an increase in back pain.

Rotation: Rotation and twisting motions are key movements in a number of sports. Twisting places increased stress on the discs of your lower spine.

Lifting: Any type of lifting can place increased stress on your spine especially when in flexion. Two important components of proper lifting techniques include keeping the object you are lifting as close to your body as possible and bending your knees while using your thigh muscles to bear as much of the weight as possible. Some sports involve more lifting than others, and you can't always follow proper lifting rules when you are playing. Bowling requires you to lift a heavy ball and swing it away from your body.

The effects of a movement can be either cumulative or acute. Cumulative means that repeating a particular motion increases its effects. Examples of cumulative effect or injury include such things as the hyperextension of a tennis serve, a wrist or forearm injury due to the bowling motion, or a low-back problem exacerbated by the repeated twisting motion of a golf swing.

An acute effect or injury is something that occurs after a single event - a quick movement outside of your normal range of motion without warming up which causes a muscle strain. An acute injury may be caused by reaching for tennis shot that is just outside your normal range, or attempting to lift a barbell weight that is beyond your physical capabilities.

Low-Risk Sports:

Bicycling, swimming, low-impact aerobics pose the least risk injury to your back.

Cycling

Whether you cycle indoors on a stationary bike or outdoors on the open road, biking is generally considered a low-risk sport relative to your back pain problem. In fact, often the advice I give to people who have jogged prior to a back injury and are finding it difficult to resume that activity is to substitute cycling.

Cycling provides you with excellent leg exercise, cardiovascular stimulation, and the experience of being outdoors without the repeated trauma to your feet, hips and knees associated with jogging or running. The only way you may irritate your back on a bicycle is by riding on a high seat and using lower handlebars so that you hyper flex your lumbar spine and place stress on the parts of your spine. Correct this position by adjusting your seat height downward so that your knee is slightly bent when at full extension on the lower pedal. If you experience sciatica pain while riding, take breaks more frequently.

Five to ten minutes on a stationary bike can be an excellent way to warm up prior to stretching and engaging in other sports.

Swimming
In general, swimming is a very safe exercise and can be excellent therapy for a back pain problem. Swimming works virtually all of your muscle in addition to providing cardiovascular conditioning. Also, being in the water protects your spine, because the buoyant properties of water help provide support and force you to move slowly and smoothly.

The type of stroke you use can increase the physical stress on your back. Strokes down on your stomach (such as the breast stroke and the crawl) are more stressful because they may place you in a position of hyperextension with your back arched. The butterfly stroke is the most irritating to your back because it requires flexing and extending. The most beneficial and safest stroke is the back stroke. As with any exercise program, warming up and stretching is important prior to beginning to swim.

Medium-Risk Sports:

Jogging and Running
The intensity of jogging or running ranges from speed walking to sprinting. The trauma as your feet hit the road transmits directly to your spine and can aggravate a lower back problem. You can do several things to minimize the impact of these forces:

Warm up and Stretch: Be sure to warm up and stretch before you start, and cool down and stretch when you finish.

Begin gradually: If you are a beginning jogger, start slowly. Start out at slower speeds and go shorter distances, until you build up your endurance and get in shape.

Wear Good Shoes: One of the most important ways to decrease the impact of road vibration to your spine is to invest in a good pair of shoes. Appropriate shoes provide excellent support for your feet as well as absorbing some of the impact to your knees, legs and lower back. A good guidance is to change your shoes every 150 miles or six months, whichever comes first.

Run on soft, smooth, flat surfaces:
Running on a grass field or gravel track is much easier on your spine than running on concrete or asphalt. Running on a flat surface causes the least amount of stress to your spine Running uphill puts your lower spine into a position of flexion because you bend forward. Running downhill also puts extra stress on your spine because you are in a posture of extension in which you arch backwards.

Racquet Sports:
Racquet sports include tennis, squash and badminton. The primary risks in all of these come from the same shots: the serve, an overhead smash, the backhand and the lunging shot to make a save.

The following are guidelines to avoid back pain problems:

Adjust your style: If you have a back pain problem, adjust your serve, overhead shots, and backhand.

Stay in shape: Stay in shape and in good overall conditioning, part of which involves allowing for an adequate warm-up time prior to playing.

Stay Warm: If you play outdoors in chilly weather, be sure to dress warmly.

Do not Lunge: The temptation to 'go for it' and get that tough shot depends on your level of competitiveness, but lunging for a shot is probably the most frequent cause of a back injury. Do not do it! Let the shot go and make up points later in the game. You'll do better overall while protecting your back.

Try Doubles: If you suffer from a severe back pain problem or are returning to a racquet sport after a back injury, consider starting out playing doubles. Doubles is easier on the back simply because you are less likely to move beyond your normal range of motion.

Wear good Shoes: Wearing good, supportive footwear when playing racquet sports helps decrease the trauma on your spine in addition to providing beneficial support for your feet.

Consider a Back Brace: If you have a chronic back problem or you are returning from a back injury, consider wearing a back brace while playing a racquet sport. A brace can provide support and protection for your back while you get in shape.

Consider your type of racquet: Consider purchasing a racquet that absorbs the most shocks when contacting the ball and provides the greatest reach.

Medium-High Risk Sports

Golf:

The twisting motion of the golf swing causes fairly significant stress on the discs and facet joints - especially if you have a tendency to arch your back extensively through the swing and try to shift your hips' through the ball' as you hit. The most common question I receive in practice is 'Can I still play golf, or when can I go back to golf'.

The following is the advice I give to these patients:

Warm up:

A proper warm up is probably the most neglected in this sport. Warming up and stretching is essential before you play.

Develop a safe swing:

Certain types of movements in a swing - such as severely arching your back as you hit the ball - can cause extra stress on your back.

Take care after long absences:

Many golfers do not get in much golfing time during the winter months. After a season of inactivity, you may be vulnerable to a back problem because your body is not properly prepared to re-enter the sport. Pay attention to proper conditioning exercises as you ease back into play.

Respect your driver and long irons:

Your back is probably most at risk when you use your driver and long irons and you are likely to utilize a full golf swing with maximum effort, putting more stress on your back. When hitting with these clubs, pay particular attention to swinging smoothly and easily. Try deciding mentally to hit the ball ten or twenty yards shorter than usual. You may actually end up hitting the ball farther and more accurately.

Wear soft-spiked shoes:

Wearing this type of shoe may actually help reduce the impact to your back at the end of your swing.

Cool Down:

After a round of golf, your body is generally limber and warm. If you jump into a car and drive home, your body cools down too rapidly without having a chance to recover from the physical demands of the game.

Take some time to hit a few short iron shots, then do some gently stretching including your neck, lower back and legs, then take a warm shower.

High Risk Sports:

Soccer & Gaelic Football:

It is difficult to do anything to make these sports more 'back friendly'. If involvement in these sports continually flares your back problem, you may want to consider some other activity.

Soccer & Gaelic Football include a variety of things such as twisting, extension, flexion and running. Try and keep all these risk factors under control by paying attention to how you approach the game: As with any sport, warm up and stretch prior to playing and be sure to play within your range of physical ability, expertise and safety relative to your back problem. You may need to adjust your level of competitiveness relative to the type of back pain problems you suffer from.

Rugby:

Rugby involves excessive twisting, hyperextension and weight bearing. It causes stress to your discs, facet joints, muscles and ligaments. If you are tackling, your back is likely flexed more than forty-five degrees and if you are being tackled, you are likely to land with your spine hyper extended or rotated If you must play, an appropriate strengthening, stretching and conditioning program is essential. You should also warm up adequately prior to playing and seriously consider wearing some type of back brace while playing.

Do not play if your back is in an acute flare-up. If you have a significant flare-up after playing be sure to have your doctor check it to determine whether you have sustained some type of significant back injury.

Chapter 11: Back to Exercise

Exercise is one of the most important treatments that can be prescribed for your back pain. Your back pain specialist will most likely prescribe a conditioning program and may add other exercises that strengthen a specific area of your back. A conditioning program will have the goals of increasing your strength, improving your flexibility, and building your endurance.

Conditioning exercises focus more on total body fitness than specific back pain, but this should always be a key component of your back pain rehabilitation program. This incorporates activities such as the exercise bike, treadmill and a walking program. A conditioning program can help you:

Manage your fear of the back pain:

Exercise requires you to move around. Beyond conditioning your body and your back, exercise reassures you that you do not have to fear your back pain or protect your movements.

Change the 'hurt equals harm' mindset:

A proper conditioning and exercise program helps you accept that increased pain does not necessarily mean injury. Your back pain may initially increase when you start to exercise, but this type of pain is often the same that non-back pain sufferers experience when they haven't worked out for a while.

Get out of the sick role:

A conditioning program also helps you address any issue that may be forcing you to maintain the sick role. If you exercise and move around, others will no longer think of you as a sick person. As they begin to treat you as a healthy person, your attitude and confidence tend to improve.

A conditioning program can be appropriate no matter what stage of back pain you have. Your back pain treatment centre specialist will prescribe a program tailored to your specific back pain problem. Your doctor should do a careful evaluation before commencing a conditioning program to ensure that you have no physical problems (such as spinal instability or fractured vertebra) that make exercise harmful. Medical problems such as heart disease or high blood pressure can also change the type of program that your back pain treatment centre specialist recommends. Do not forget to tell your doctor and specialist if you are on any medications or if you are pregnant.

Your pain may initially increase:

When you begin the program, you will be using muscles that you've probably been protecting for a while. As a result, you may experience a mild to moderate increase in pain. This pain does not mean that you are injuring your back, and that initial pain should decrease over time.

You must be willing to follow the program independently:

Your back pain treatment centre specialist will probably monitor you closely at the beginning of the program and then instruct you to go ahead and complete the exercise on your own. To really conquer your pain, you must be willing to follow through with the program on your own.

You must comply with the conditioning recommendations:

Cutting the conditioning exercises short can be very tempting, DO NOT!

Back pain has different phases. Your conditioning program depends on which phase you are experiencing, with chronic back pain, your muscles may be weak from inactivity. Your conditioning program will start out slowly and build in intensity over time.

Initial Phase of acute back pain (one to five days)

Your pain and muscle spasms may be limiting during this phase. Ice, bed rest and some gentle knee to chest stretches on day two to five.

Acute back pain (less than one month's duration)

Mild exercise that you gradually increase can help you avoid the next stage of back pain altogether. Mild exercise, such as limited walking is appropriate. Over the next several weeks, you can slowly add more strenuous activities such as faster walking, swimming or bicycling. At this stage of treatment avoid any severe twisting or bending motions. Let your pain be your guide - exercise until you experience more pain and then stop at that point.

Sub-acute back pain (one to three months duration)

Exercise and conditioning issues become very important in this phase. Try to keep as active as possible, even with ongoing back pain. Exercises may initially increase your pain but those in this book are designed to be safe for your spine.

Chronic Back Pain (longer than three month's duration)

At this stage, a physical reconditioning program that includes strengthening, stretching and aerobics should be part of your total treatment plan. As you begin to use the weakened muscles, your back pain initially will increase. Slowly work through the pain by completing a certain number of repetitions regardless of the pain.

Recurrent acute back pain (pain flare-ups with pain-free episodes in between)

Participating in an aerobic conditioning exercise program three times per week can significantly decrease the frequency, intensity and duration of your back pain episodes. It must include aerobic, stretching and strengthening elements.

The aerobic component can be anything from speed walking to the exercise bike to the treadmill. Even though aerobic exercise is not targeted directly at your back, this type of exercise helps you manage your back pain more effectively, improve your mental abilities, provide stress relief and help you sleep better.

Quota System:

The quota system is a specialized approach to your exercise program. You work to a specific quota rather than being guided by your pain. Exercising in this way is especially important if you are in the sub-acute and chronic stages of back pain.

To set up a quota system for any exercise, begin by establishing your baseline. Your baseline for that exercise is the amount of exercise you can do until either pain or fatigue stops you. Your amount of exercise can be measured in several ways depending upon the type of exercise (the time it takes, number of repetitions or distance).

Record this figure for three consecutive exercise sessions to get a good measure of your baseline capabilities For example: You can do your treadmill exercise for five minutes on the first session, six minutes on the second session and seven minutes on the third session. In each of these sessions you would have stopped when the pain or fatigue became uncomfortable. In this example you take the average of the three sessions to establish your baseline of six minutes (5 + 6 + 7 = 18, divide by 3 to get 6). After you establish the baseline, subtract 20 percent. The remaining number sets your initial quota. In this example, 6 - 20% = 4.8. Your initial quota, then is roughly five minutes,

After you establish your initial quota, you complete that goal regardless of your back pain. You then set increasing quotas for yourself based on discussions with your back pain treatment centre specialist. One example may be to increase your quota by 10 percent each week or every third exercise session.

You can use the quota system for any of your exercises or activities: The distance you can walk, lengths you can swim, amount of time you can sit at a desk, and time on the treadmill. The important point to remember about quotas is that the goal is to work to the quota rather than pain. Do not make your quotas too difficult or potentially unachievable. If you can't achieve a particular quota, simply reduce it a little for a couple of sessions and then return to your previous quota goals.

Pacing:

Pacing your activities involves a gradual increase in activity according to a specific plan. This concept also involves taking an extensive activity and breaking it up into smaller pieces (with breaks in between) to help prevent any flare-up in your back pain problem.

Pacing your activities prevents a common pattern that involves overdoing and crashing. You may experience the overdoing and crashing pattern if you vigorously engage in an activity when your back pain is minimal only to have it cause a flare-up that sets you back.

Pacing involves doing a reasonable amount of exercise or activity, with breaks in between so that you keep your back pain under reasonable control.

Set aside time to Exercise:

Plan ahead. Make sure you can be private and undisturbed

during your exercise time. Your exercise routine should take from fifteen to thirty minutes to complete and be done three to five times per week. Alternate your back exercise program and aerobic conditioning every other day. If you choose to exercise in the morning, it is a good idea to walk around first after getting up before doing your back exercises.

Exercise on a firm but comfortable surface and wear loose-fitting clothing:

Carpet or exercise mats provide a good exercise surface. Do not do your exercises on a very soft surface such as a bed or couch. Soft surfaces do not provide your body or your back with adequate support to do the exercises safely.

Move slowly and smoothly:

Especially when you are starting this type of exercise program, concentrate on making your movements easy and graceful. Take a brief rest between each exercise if you find that helps you complete the program.

Progress at your own pace:

When beginning an exercise regime, do the number of repetitions that cause you little, if any, discomfort. Increase your repetitions using the quota system. Start out with two or three repetitions of a particular exercise and add one repetition per week until you reach your goal.

At no point during your back exercise program should you feel that you are straining beyond what you feel are your physical capabilities or to the point of significantly increasing your pain.

Focus on your breathing:

Try to breathe evenly and deeply. Avoid holding your breath or taking shallow breaths. A good technique to ensure healthy breathing is to inhale slowly through your nose and exhale slowly though your mouth.

Exercise Warnings:

See your doctor if you experience numbness in the genital area or muscle weakness in your legs.

Do not start your exercise program in the middle of an acute attack.

The waiting period may be anywhere from one day to three weeks after onset of pain.

Expect some soreness and discomfort.

Muscles will naturally be sore after you start exercising them. If at any time you experience a dramatic increase in pain, or any new type of pain, see your doctor.

PART 1:

Initial

Phase:

Commence from day 5 to day 21 since onset of Back Pain.

EXERCISE 1:
KEEP MOVING AND MOBILE

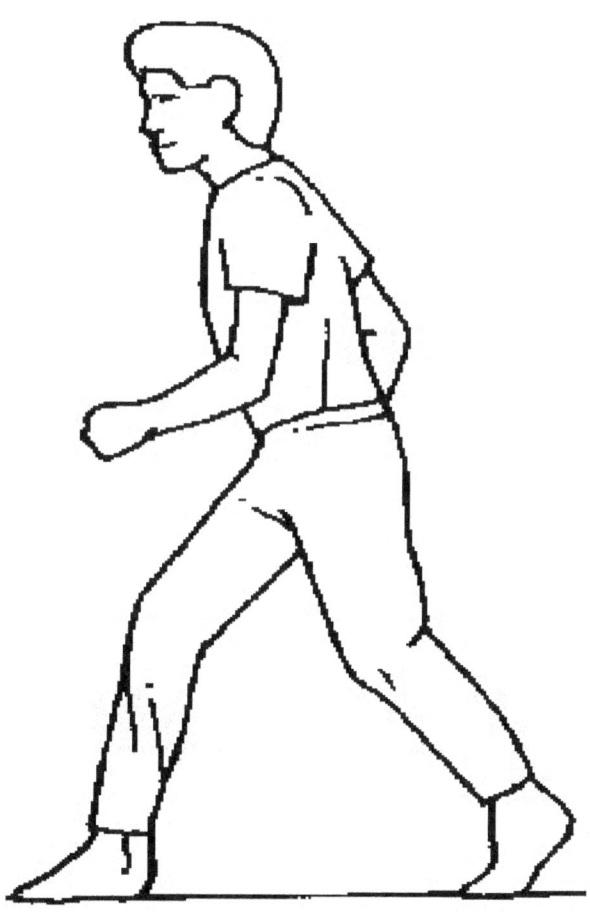

Walk for twenty minutes on a flat surface at a comfortable pace. Try and note the distance you have walked in the twenty minutes. Make a note of it and then use the quota system as described in previous chapter.

EXERCISE 2
KEEP ACTIVE:

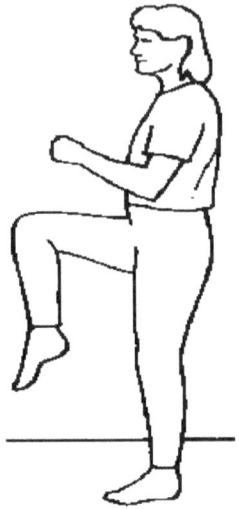

March in place for sixty seconds. Take a break for sixty seconds. March again for sixty seconds. Preferably do in front of a mirror and a clock.

EXERCISE 3:
KNEE ROLLING:

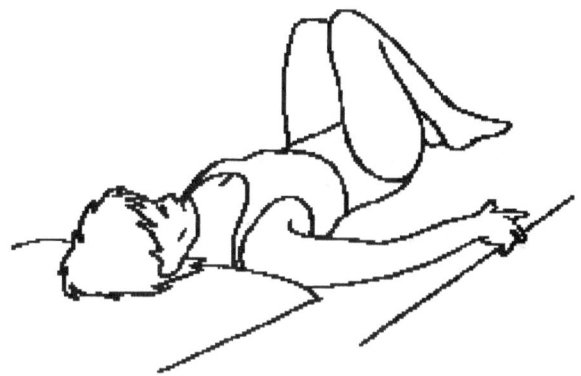

Lying on your back with knees together and bent.

Slowly roll your knees from side to side keeping your upper trunk still.

Repeat twenty times.

EXERCISE 4:
ROTATION:

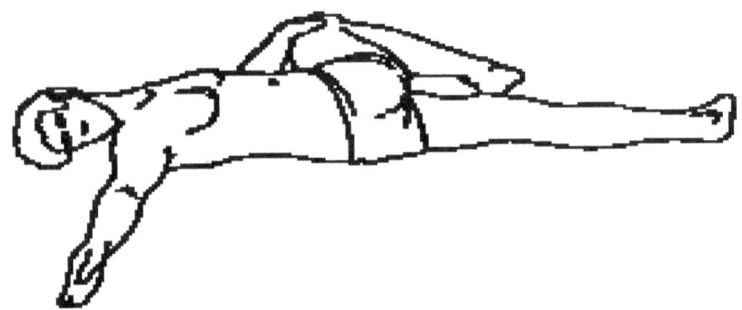

Lying on your back with one leg bent.

Bring your bent knee over the other leg and push your knee against the floor with the opposite hand. Then reach with the other arm to the opposite side looking in the same direction. You will feel the stretching in your lower back and bottom. Hold approx. 20 secs. - relax.

Repeat three to five times.

PART 2: Sub- Acute Phase:

Commence from day 21 to day 41 since onset of Back Pain.

EXERCISE 1:
KNEE ROLLING:

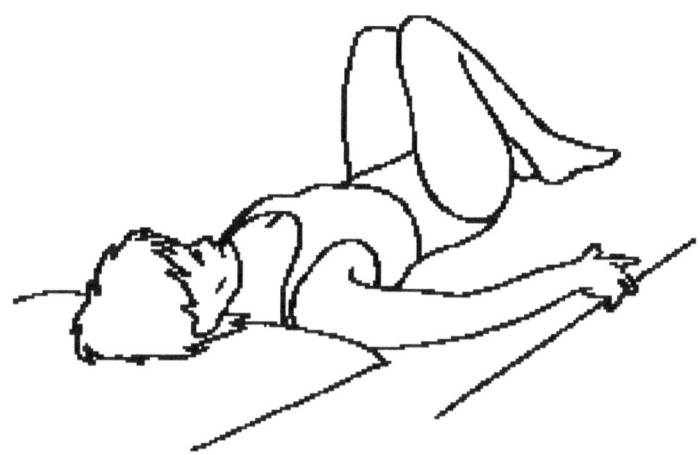

Lying on your back with knees together and bent.

Slowly roll your knees from side to side keeping your upper trunk still.

Repeat twenty times.

EXERCISE 2:
ROTATION:

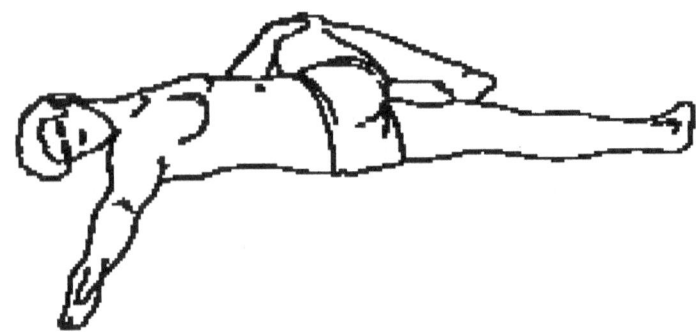

Lying on your back with one leg bent.

Bring your bent knee over the other leg and push your knee against the floor with the opposite hand.

Then reach with the other arm to the opposite side looking in the same direction. You will feel the stretching in your lower back and bottom. Hold approx. 20 secs. - relax.

Repeat three to five times.

EXERCISE 3:
PELVIC LIFT:

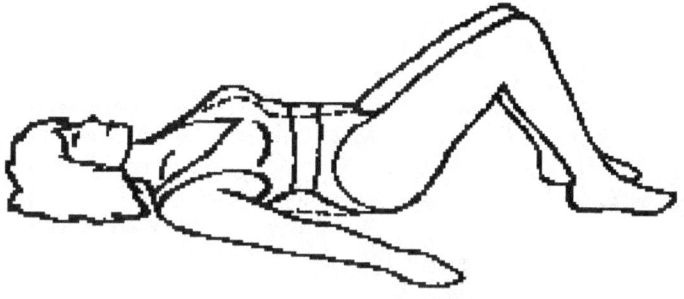

Tighten your stomach muscles by pushing your back down and curving your bottom up - relax.

Continue the exercise by pushing your bottom down and tightening your back muscles to arch your lumbar (lower) spine up - relax.

Repeat five times.

EXERCISE 4:
PARTIAL SIT-UP

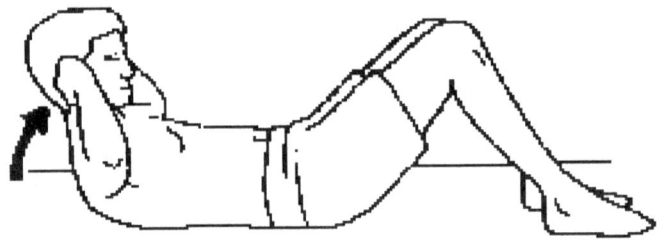

PARTIAL SIT-UP

Lying on your back with your fingers just behind your ears and elbows out.

Tighten your stomach muscles and lift your head and shoulders off the floor.

Repeat five times.

EXERCISE 5:
HAMSTRING STRETCH:

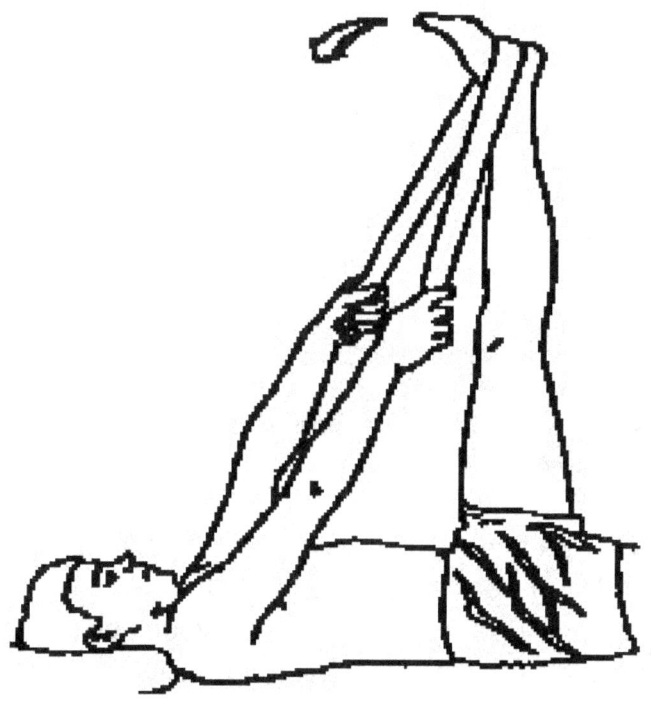

Lying on your back with a cushion under your head. Put a band under the sole of your foot and hold onto the band with both hands.

Lift your leg straight up. Pull the band flexing the ankle and stretching the back of your thigh. Hold approx. 20 secs. - relax.

Repeat three to five times

EXERCISE 6:
CAT AND CAMEL

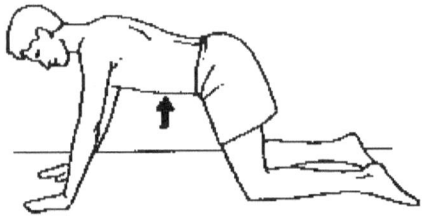

CAT AND CAMEL:

This exercise is designed to strengthen your back and abdominal muscles.

1. Start on your hands and knees with your weight evenly distributed and your neck parallel to the floor.
2. Arch your back upward by tightening your abdominal and buttock muscles, letting your head drop slightly.
3. Hold for a count of five.
4. Let your back sag gently toward the floor, while keeping your arms straight.
Keep your weight evenly distributed between your legs and arms
5. Hold for a count of five again.
Do two or three repetitions initially and work your way up to five repetitions.
Be sure to make your movements slow and smooth.
Inhale through your nose as you arch your back and exhale through your mouth as you let your back sag.

EXERCISE 7:
WALL SLIDE

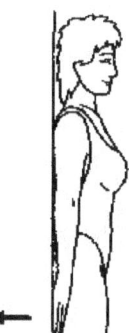

- Stand with your back against a wall and feet shoulder width apart.
- Place your hands on your hips or let your arms hang at your sides, whichever is more comfortable.

- Keep your head level by focusing directly in front of you.

- Slide smoothly down the wall into a crouched position with your knees bent to ninety degrees.

- If you have trouble going down this far, slide down half way.
- Hold this position for a count of five.
- Slide smoothly up to your starting position.
- Initially you may be only able to complete two or three repetitions of this exercise. Your goal is to complete five repetitions while holding the crouched position for one minute each time. Work up to this goal gradually.

EXERCISE 8:
SIDE STRETCH

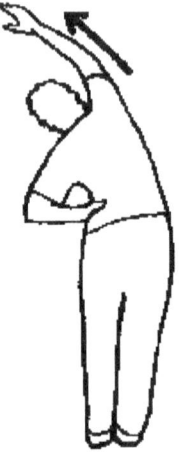

1. Stretch one arm over your head and bend your upper body to the opposite side.
2. Put your other hand on your waist and do not twist your body as you bend.
3. Hold the stretch for a count of five.
4. Return to the starting position with your hands and arms at your sides.
5. Repeat this movement five times.
6. Switch to the other side and repeat steps 1 to 5.
This exercise stretches the muscles of your back and sides.

PART 3:

ADVANCED ROUTINE:

Commence from 6 weeks since onset of Back Pain.

EXERCISE 1:
PELVIC TILT

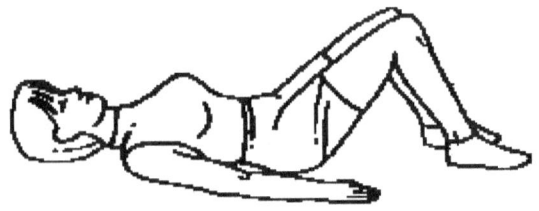

Lying on your back with knees bent.

Flatten the small of your back against the floor.

Hold for five to ten seconds.

Repeat three times.

EXERCISE 2:
Single and Double Leg Pull

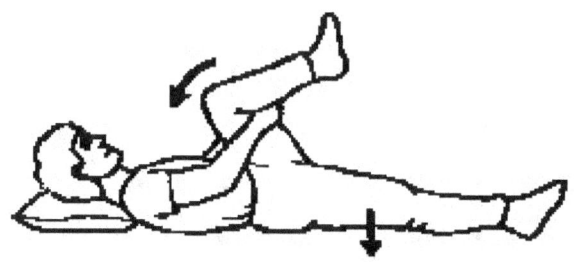

SINGLE AND DOUBLE LEG PULL

Lying on your back with a cushion under your head.

Pull your knee onto your stomach helping with your hands. Push your other leg down towards the floor.

Hold approx. 20 secs. - relax.

Repeat five times.

Switch legs and repeat again five times.

DOUBLE LEG PULL.

Pull both knees onto your stomach helping with your hands. Hold for twenty seconds.

EXERCISE 3:
KNEE ROLLING:

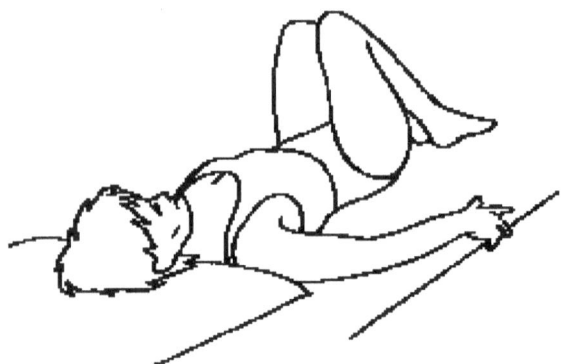

Lying on your back with knees together and bent.

Slowly roll your knees from side to side keeping your upper trunk still.

Repeat twenty times.

EXERCISE 4:
ROTATION:

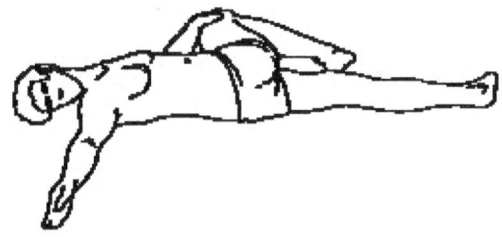

Lying on your back with one leg bent.

Bring your bent knee over the other leg and push your knee against the floor with the opposite hand.

Then reach with the other arm to the opposite side looking in the same direction.

You will feel the stretching in your lower back and bottom. Hold approx. 20 secs. - relax.

Repeat three to five times.

EXERCISE 5:
PELVIC LIFT:

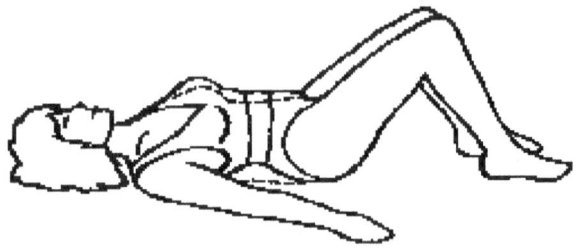

Tighten your stomach muscles by pushing your back down and curving your bottom up - relax.

Continue the exercise by pushing your bottom down and tightening your back muscles to arch your lumbar (lower) spine up - relax.

Repeat five times.

EXERCISE 6:
PARTIAL SIT-UP

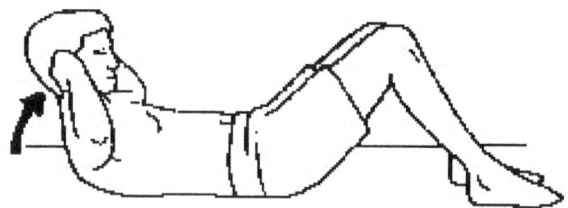

PARTIAL SIT-UP

Lying on your back with your fingers just behind your ears and elbows out.

Tighten your stomach muscles and lift your head and shoulders off the floor.

Repeat five times.

EXERCISE 7:
OBLIQUE SIT-UP

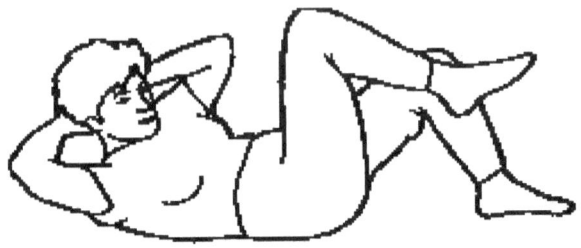

OBLIQUE SIT-UP

Lying on your back with knees bent and hands clasped behind your neck.

Lift your upper trunk by bringing your chin towards your chest and tightening your stomach muscles, then reach with your elbow towards your opposite knee letting the knee come up a bit. Return to starting position. Repeat with other side.

Repeat three to five times for each side.

EXERCISE 8:
HAMSTRING STRETCH:

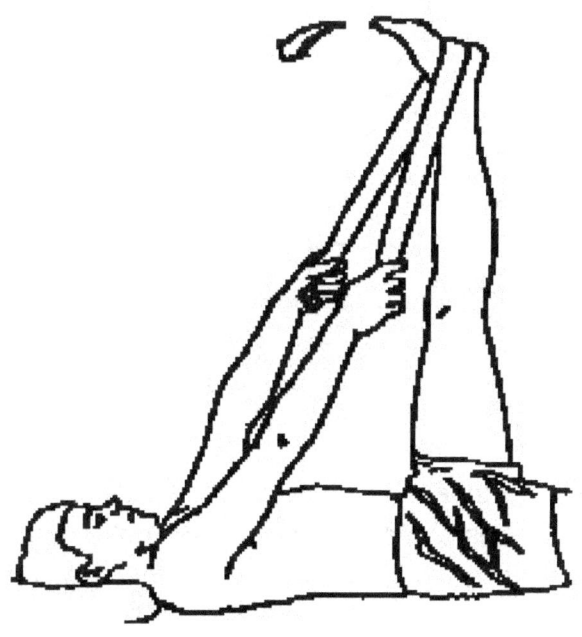

Lying on your back with a cushion under your head. Put a band under the sole of your foot and hold onto the band with both hands.

Lift your leg straight up. Pull the band flexing the ankle and stretching the back of your thigh. Hold approx. 20 secs. - relax.

Repeat three to five times.

EXERCISE 9:
THE PUSH UP

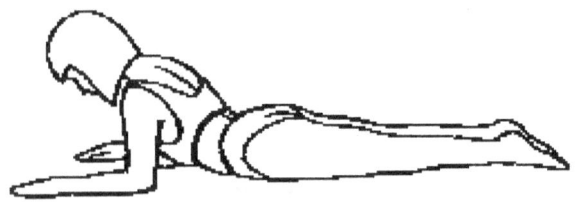

This exercise stretches the muscles of your abdominal area and provides some upper body strengthening.

1. Lie on your stomach with your feet slightly apart, place your face near the floor or rest your forehead on the floor, and your hands palm-down at face level.

2. Use your arms to gradually push the top half of your body to a resting position on your elbows.

You may feel tightness in your lower back or abdomen. Try to hold this position for 20 seconds or more until you feel comfortable.

3. Push up with your arms (with your hands on the floor) as high as possible while keeping your hips and legs flat on the floor).

Remember to keep your back relaxed.

4. Hold the position for 20 to 30 seconds.

5. Slowly lower yourself back to the floor.

Initially, do two or three repetitions, and work your way up to about five repetitions.

EXERCISE 10:
CAT AND CAMEL

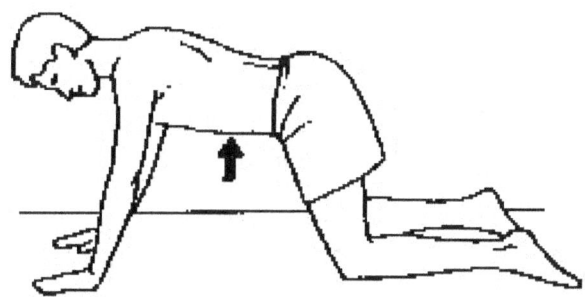

CAT AND CAMEL:
This exercise is designed to strengthen your back and abdominal muscles.

1. Start on your hands and knees with your weight evenly distributed and your neck parallel to the floor.

2. Arch your back upward by tightening your abdominal and buttock muscles, letting your head drop slightly.

3. Hold for a count of five.

4. Let your back sag gently toward the floor, while keeping your arms straight.
Keep your weight evenly distributed between your legs and arms

5. Hold for a count of five again.
Do two or three repetitions initially and work your way up to five repetitions. Be sure to make your movements slow and smooth.
Inhale through your nose as you arch your back and exhale through your mouth as you let your back sag.

EXERCISE 11:
ARM STRETCH:

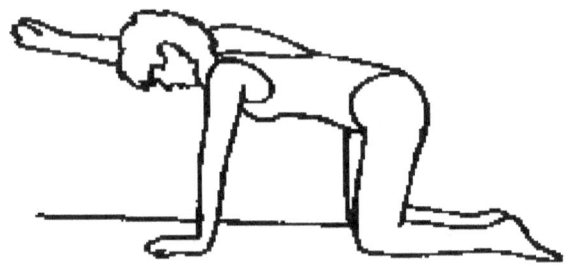

ARM REACH

This exercise is designed to strengthen the muscles of your shoulders and upper back.

1. Start on your hands and knees with your weight evenly distributed and your neck parallel to the floor.

2. Stretch out one arm in front of you being careful not to raise your head.

Keep your weight evenly distributed between your knees and one arm on the floor.

3. Hold the arm reach for a count of five.

4. Return to the starting position.

5. Do five repetitions with the same arm.

6. Switch to your other arm and repeat steps 2 through 5.

EXERCISE 12:
LEG REACH

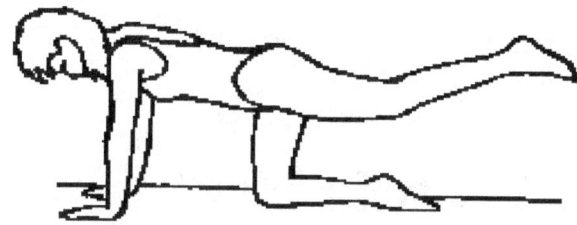

LEG REACH

This exercise is designed to strengthen the muscles of your buttocks.

1. Start on your hands and knees with your weight evenly distributed and your neck parallel to the floor.

2. Slowly extend one leg straight out behind you and hold it parallel to the floor.
Your foot may be pointed or flexed - whichever is comfortable for you.
As you extend your leg, do not let your back, head or stomach sag.
Make sure no one is behind you when you do this move!
3. Hold this position for a count of five.
You may only be able to hold this position for two or three seconds when you start out. This is typical when first practicing this exercise and your endurance will improve as you gain strength and stability through practice.
4. Return to the starting position and repeat this movement three to five times.
5. Switch legs and repeat steps 2, 3 and 4.

EXERCISE 13:
ALTERNATE ARM AND LEG REACH

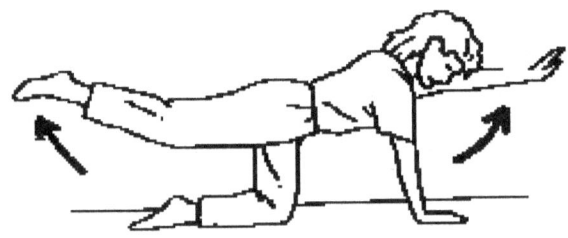

1. Start on your hands and knees with your weight evenly distributed and your neck parallel to the floor.

2. Extend one leg backward, parallel to the floor and at the same time reach forward with the opposite arm.

Try to make your leg, torso, head and arm form a straight line parallel to the floor.

3. Hold this position for a count of three.

4. Lower your leg and arm to the starting position.

5. Repeat the same movements with your other side.

Work your way up to five repetitions of this exercise on each side.

The alternate arm and leg reach helps strengthen your shoulders, upper back and buttocks.

EXERCISE 14:
WALL SLIDE

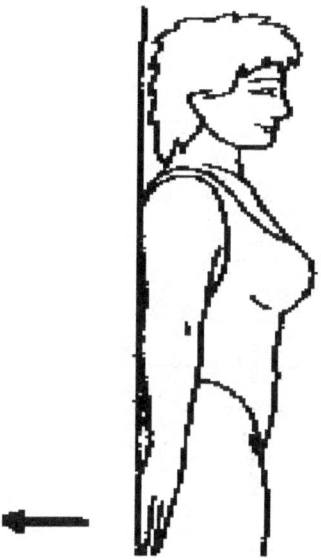

Stand with your back against a wall and feet shoulder width apart.

Place your hands on your hips or let your arms hang at your sides, whichever is more comfortable.
Keep your head level by focusing directly in front of you.
Slide smoothly down the wall into a crouched position with your knees bent to ninety degrees.

If you have trouble going down this far, slide down half way.

Hold this position for a count of five.
Slide smoothly up to your starting position.

Initially you may be only able to complete two or three repetitions of this exercise. Your goal is to complete five repetitions while holding the crouched position for one minute each time. Work up to this goal gradually.

EXERCISE 15:
SIDE STRETCH

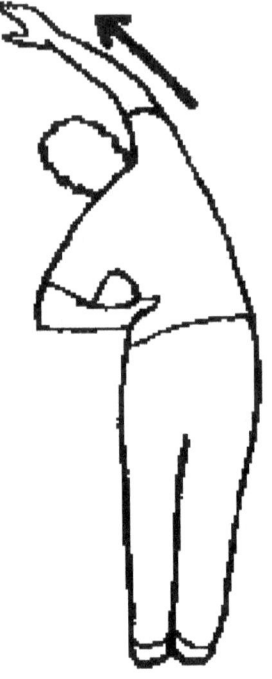

1. Stretch one arm over your head and bend your upper body to the opposite side.

2. Put your other hand on your waist and do not twist your body as you bend.

3. Hold the stretch for a count of five.

4. Return to the starting position with your hands and arms at your sides.
5. Repeat this movement five times.
6. Switch to the other side and repeat steps 1 to 5.

This exercise stretches the muscles of your back and sides.

EXERCISE 16:
BACK ARCH

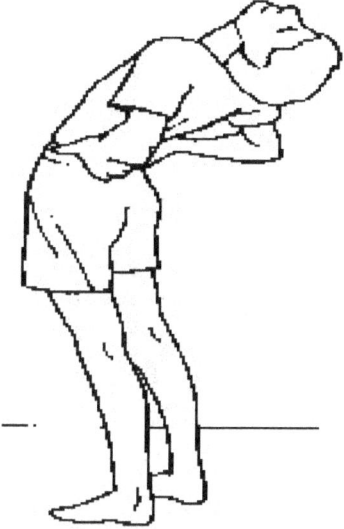

Stand up straight with feet shoulder width apart and pointing directly forward.

Place the palms of your hands on your lower back.

Gently breathe in and out until you feel relaxed.

Support your back with your hands while bending your back as far backwards as possible. Keep your knees straight during the exercise.
The back arch stretches your shoulder, back and hip muscles.
Try exhaling (breathing out) as you lean back.
Hold the arch for a count of five.

Gradually return to your starting position.

Repeat three to five times.

Conclusion:

Most effective therapeutic interventions are given as a course during which the effects of the treatment accumulate.

Second and subsequent treatments are guided by the response to earlier treatments.

Most frequently you will have noted some benefit after the first treatment but it probably did not last. The intensity of the treatment is slightly increased to achieve cumulative benefit for more profound and longer-lasting effects. It is not uncommon for patients not to respond until after they have had the six sessions.

There is no such thing as a quick fix. If you sprained your ankle, you would not expect to be miraculously cured after one magical treatment. The back is a part of your body and takes time to repair.

After fifteen years and having treated over 7,000 backs in both private and public settings in Ireland and the USA, I began to research why some people did not recover.

Ninety-seven per cent of my patients responded well and were delighted with the outcome but three per cent did not.

I studied their files to understand why they were different, and did they share any common features.

Most of them did.

The majority of those that didn't respond never followed the plan, they dropped out before the sixth session, they did not undertake the exercise program, they did not follow any of the back care advice. They did not help themselves.

You owe it to yourself to be one of the ninety-seven percent. Stick to the treatment plan, follow the advice, do the exercises and conquer your pain.

I wish you a safe and successful journey.

Duncan